Contents

Colour plates are to be found between pp. 118 and 119.

Contributors

Dilly O. C. Anumba MBBS FWACS FRCOG MD LL.M (Medical Law)
Professor of Obstetrics and Gynaecology, the University of Sheffield, and Honorary Consultant Obstetrician and Gynaecologist, Subspecialist in Fetomaternal Medicine, at the Department of Obstetrics and Gynaecology, Sheffield Teaching Hospitals NHS Foundation Trust, Sheffield, UK

Julia F. Bodle MD MRCOG DipMedEd
Consultant Obstetrician and Gynaecologist at the Department of Obstetrics and Gynaecology, Sheffield Teaching Hospitals NHS Foundation Trust, Sheffield, UK

Fiona M. Fairlie MD FRCOG
Consultant Obstetrician and Gynaecologist at the Department of Obstetrics and Gynaecology, Sheffield Teaching Hospitals NHS Foundation Trust, Sheffield, UK

Frances Hills MRCOG
Specialty Trainee, East Midlands (North), Nottingham, UK

Chibuike Godson Ikeri Iruloh MBBS MRCOG PhD
Consultant Obstetrician and Gynaecologist, Subspecialist in Fetomaternal Medicine, at the Department of Obstetrics and Gynaecology, St Mary's Hospital, Central Manchester University Hospitals NHS Foundation Trust, Manchester, UK

Swati Jha MD FRCOG
Consultant Obstetrician and Gynaecologist at the Department of Obstetrics and Gynaecology, Sheffield Teaching Hospitals NHS Foundation Trust, and Honorary Senior Clinical Lecturer, University of Sheffield, Sheffield, UK

Shehnaaz Jivraj MBChB MD MRCOG
Consultant Obstetrician and Gynaecologist at the Department of Obstetrics and Gynaecology, Sheffield Teaching Hospitals NHS Foundation Trust, Sheffield, UK

Remon Keriakos MBBS FRCOG
Consultant Obstetrician and Gynaecologist at the Department of Obstetrics and Gynaecology, Sheffield Teaching Hospitals NHS Foundation Trust, Sheffield, UK

Madeleine MacDonald MBChB(Hons) MRCOG PGCert (Medical Leadership)
Specialty Trainee in Obstetrics and Gynaecology at the Department of Obstetrics and Gynaecology, Sheffield Teaching Hospitals NHS Foundation Trust, Sheffield, UK

Priya Madhuvrata MD MRCOG
Consultant Obstetrician and Gynaecologist at the Department of Obstetrics and Gynaecology, Sheffield Teaching Hospitals NHS Foundation Trust, Sheffield, UK

Nusrat Mir BSc(Hons) MBChB MRCGP MRCPsych
Consultant in Perinatal Psychiatry and Honorary Senior Lecturer, Perinatal Mental Health Service, Michael Carlisle Centre, Sheffield, UK

Meena Srinivas MD MRCOG
Consultant Obstetrician and Gynaecologist at Barnsley District General Hospital, Barnsley, UK

Victoria Stern MBChB BSc MRCOG
Clinical Research Fellow at the Academic Unit of Developmental and Reproductive Medicine, University of Sheffield, Sheffield, UK

Sarah Vause MD FRCOG
Consultant Obstetrician, Subspecialist in Fetomaternal Medicine, at the Department of Obstetrics and Gynaecology, St Mary's Hospital, Central Manchester University Hospitals NHS Foundation Trust, Manchester, UK

Hannah Yeeles MRCOG
Specialty Trainee in Obstetrics and Gynaecology at the Department of Obstetrics and Gynaecology, Sheffield Teaching Hospitals NHS Foundation Trust, Sheffield, UK

Antenatal Disorders for the MRCOG and Beyond

Second Edition

Antenatal Disorders for the MRCOG and Beyond

Second Edition

Edited by Dilly Anumba and Shehnaaz Jivraj

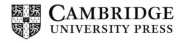

CAMBRIDGE
UNIVERSITY PRESS

CAMBRIDGE
UNIVERSITY PRESS

University Printing House, Cambridge CB2 8BS, United Kingdom

Cambridge University Press is part of the University of Cambridge.

It furthers the University's mission by disseminating knowledge in the pursuit of education, learning and research at the highest international levels of excellence.

www.cambridge.org
Information on this title: www.cambridge.org/9781107684928

First published: 2000, the Royal College of Obstetricians and Gynaecologists

Second edition 2016

Printed in the United Kingdom by Clays, St. Ives plc

A catalogue record for this publication is available from the British Library

Library of Congress Cataloguing in Publication data
Names: Anumba, Dilly, editor. | Jivraj, Shehnaaz, editor. | Thomson, Andrew J. (Andrew John).
Antenatal disorders for the MRCOG and beyond. Preceded by (work):
Title: Antenatal disorders for the MRCOG and beyond / edited by Dilly Anumba
and Shehnaaz Jivraj.
Description: Second edition. | Cambridge, United Kingdom ; New York : Cambridge University
Press, 2016. | Preceded by Antenatal disorders for the MRCOG and beyond / Andrew J. Thomson,
Ian A. Greer. London : RCOG, 2000. | Includes bibliographical references and index.
Identifiers: LCCN 2015040093 | ISBN 9781107684928 (Paperback : alk. paper)
Subjects: | MESH: Pregnancy Complications–diagnosis. | Pregnancy
Complications–therapy. | Prenatal Care–methods.
Classification: LCC RG551 | NLM WQ 240 | DDC 618.2–dc23 LC record available at
http://lccn.loc.gov/2015040093

ISBN 978-1-107-68492-8 Paperback

Preface

Antenatal care has evolved in line with advances in screening, diagnosis and management of maternal and fetal conditions. The core objective of such care has remained the same, namely to provide support for the pregnant woman that should culminate in the safe birth of a healthy baby to a healthy mother. Antenatal care is increasingly underpinned by an evidence base of clinical effectiveness that also increasingly dispels traditional myths of care philosophies and interventions with no evidence of benefit. Central to this evolution has remained the need to categorize care in such a way that pregnancies with identified risk factors are provided with additional support while those with few or no identifiable risk factors are provided with a care package that does not involve undue medicalization. A team approach that involves midwives working, when required, with obstetricians, physicians and social support services is now recognized to provide the most composite package of care that adapts flexibly to what the pregnant woman requires. Community-based care, often in the woman's home, with hospital visits when necessary, has become the preferred approach to antenatal service delivery. Better understanding of medical disorders of pregnancy, and more sensitive screening approaches, inform the approaches to antenatal care outlined in this book. As with the first edition, this volume will prove extremely valuable to anyone, not only in the UK but also in other countries, striving to provide the best possible care for pregnant women.

Dilly Anumba and Shehnaaz Jivraj

1 Antenatal care and risk assessment

Dilly Anumba

Introduction

Pregnancy is a physiological process during which most women remain well and require very little medical input. However, some women develop complications with significant morbidity or mortality for their baby and, occasionally, for themselves. Providers of antenatal care must be able to distinguish between these two groups of women and arrange with them an appropriate and personalized plan of care. Such a care plan could range from the simple, with no requirement for complex investigations and care, to the more challenging, requiring substantial medical expertise to enable adequate monitoring of the mother and the fetus. The purpose of antenatal care is to support the pregnant mother through her birth experience and to distinguish the normal from the at-risk pregnancy, identifying pregnancy risk factors and stratifying care to improve the chances of a successful pregnancy culminating in a healthy outcome.

Epidemiological and observational studies have demonstrated that women who receive antenatal care have better pregnancy outcomes, with lower maternal and perinatal mortality, than those who do not. These studies have also demonstrated an association between the number of antenatal visits and pregnancy outcomes after controlling for confounding factors such as the length of gestation.

Patterns and provision of antenatal care have changed enormously in recent years in response to the opinions of consumers, providers and professional associations, and government reports. The Department of Health's *Changing Childbirth* and *Maternity Matters* reports highlighted the need for women to be the focus of maternity care, with an emphasis on providing choice, easy access and continuity of care.[1,2] Pregnant women should be provided with care that enables them to make informed decisions about their options. Good antenatal care should focus on those practices that have been shown to be effective and have a favourable impact on maternal and fetal outcomes.

Antenatal Disorders for the MRCOG and Beyond, Second Edition, ed. Dilly Anumba and Shehnaaz Jivraj. Published by Cambridge University Press. © Cambridge University Press 2016.

What is the purpose of antenatal care?

The aim of antenatal care is to provide support for the pregnant mother and her family, which should culminate in a safe birth and recovery. In order to achieve this, the following care objectives should be met during this period:

- To provide advice, reassurance, education and support for the woman and her family.
- To deal with the minor ailments of pregnancy, such as abdominal discomfort, heartburn, backache, haemorrhoids, nausea and vomiting and varicose veins.
- To screen for, diagnose and manage pre-existing maternal disorders, such as diabetes, heart disease and infection. Screening for such conditions should continue until the end of pregnancy to confirm that women who screen negative at the beginning remain well throughout.
- To promptly identify and treat any new medical or obstetric problems arising in pregnancy, and, where possible, to prevent these from adversely affecting the health of the mother or her baby.
- To plan for labour and delivery, care of the newborn and future general and reproductive health.

Antenatal risk assessment

Defining the risk of adverse pregnancy outcome posed by identifiable clinical factors can help stratify and plan antenatal care for individual women. Risk assessment has underpinned the provision of antenatal care for several decades and can inform categorization into scores that determine clinical care. Applying this concept to antenatal care, Alexander and Keirse evaluated formal antenatal risk scoring for perinatal mortality, preterm delivery, intrauterine growth restriction and low Apgar score at birth.[3] They found that risk scoring performed poorly in identifying women at risk of these conditions. One reason for this observation may have been the well-known fact that screening is more effective in multiparous than nulliparous women, partly attributable to the fact that most risk markers are based on events in previous pregnancies. For risk scoring to be beneficial in antenatal care, the component factors need to have high predictive values for the adverse pregnancy outcome that they are anticipated to predict. If this is not the case, then risk scoring may result in more harm than good. Women who are labelled as being at increased risk of an adverse outcome may suffer unnecessary stress and anxiety and will be exposed to unnecessary investigations and interventions, some of which may be deleterious to the pregnancy at substantial avoidable cost to the taxpayer.

Despite the limitations of pregnancy risk scoring, assessing risk broadly can inform the care plan outlined at the beginning of antenatal care.

Assessing women for clinical risks should happen before pregnancy, throughout pregnancy, and in labour, as risk factors can change at any time during gestation, sometimes necessitating a change in care plan and intervention to mitigate those risks. One study that evaluated risk scoring during pregnancy showed that while 96% of primigravidae were considered low risk in early pregnancy, only 39% remained low risk by the end of pregnancy, 57% having developed risk factors during pregnancy or labour. Similarly, 74% of multigravidae were categorized as low risk at booking, but by the end of labour only 48% remained low risk.[4] Since unidentified risk factors will arise during pregnancy and the majority of women will have required some form of obstetric input by the time they give birth, the value of formal risk scoring in early pregnancy has been questioned. Nevertheless, risk assessment at the beginning of pregnancy enables those women with risk factors for adverse pregnancy outcome to be identified early for appropriate referrals, so that those without identifiable risk factors can be deemed suitable for midwife/general practitioner antenatal care. For the latter group, locally agreed protocols, informed by national guidance where possible, should be established for the identification, referral and treatment of obstetric complications.

The common clinical conditions that are currently screened for during pregnancy are outlined below, in the section on the booking visit. In addition to those conditions for which supportive research evidence for screening exists, there are several pregnancy conditions that are not currently screened for routinely. It could prove reasonable to screen for some of these conditions routinely in the future if supportive research evidence, expert or consensus opinion or favourable cost–benefit considerations evolve.

Who should see women at antenatal visits, and where?

While the first antenatal contact with the pregnant woman should happen at her home or in a primary care facility such as the general practitioner (GP) surgery, and should usually be provided by the designated midwife, the formal booking clinic may be provided at the hospital, when, depending on the presence of any pregnancy risk factors, the woman may require to see an obstetrician as well. Furthermore, a hospital booking visit may enable the simultaneous conduct of ultrasound scan examinations and the performance of antenatal screening tests which may not have been feasible in the community for logistic reasons or because of gestational timing. Pregnancies not associated with any significant identifiable risk factors may then be followed up by community-based visits coordinated by the midwife or GP. Those pregnancies with risk factors that warrant obstetric input may require to be supervised by the obstetrician through regular hospital visits alternating with community-based care by the named designated midwife. Care is optimized when antenatal care is provided by a named group of professionals with whom the pregnant mother develops rapport and trust.

Antenatal interventions which are not routinely recommended

Antenatal care has traditionally involved many routine interventions with little or no research evidence of benefit. Such routine care interventions of no proven benefit include: repeated maternal weighing, breast or pelvic examination, iron or vitamin A supplementation, and routine screening for chlamydia, cytomegalovirus, hepatitis C virus, group B streptococcus, toxoplasmosis and bacterial vaginosis. The routine use of Doppler ultrasound to monitor low-risk uncomplicated pregnancies, ultrasound estimation of fetal size for suspected large-for-gestational-age unborn babies, and screening for gestational diabetes using fasting plasma glucose, random blood glucose, glucose challenge test or urinalysis are of no proven benefit. Similarly, routine fetal-movement counting, auscultation of the fetal heart, antenatal electronic cardiotocography and routine ultrasound scanning after 24 weeks have no supportive evidence of benefit in routine care of uncomplicated pregnancies.

Who should provide antenatal care?

In recent years, there has been much debate concerning the issue of which of the care professionals involved with delivering maternity services should provide antenatal care. A study carried out in Scotland in 1989 showed that obstetricians, general practitioners and midwives working together (shared care) provided 97% of antenatal care.[5] A review of published patterns of care by the National Institute for Health and Care Excellence (NICE) recently concluded that midwife- and GP-led models of care should be offered to women with an uncomplicated pregnancy, highlighting that the routine involvement of obstetricians in the care of these women at scheduled times does not appear to improve perinatal outcomes, compared with involving obstetricians only when complications arise.[6] Care should be provided continuously throughout the antenatal period by a small group of healthcare professionals with whom the woman feels comfortable. However, there should be clear referral paths to appropriate specialist teams for women who require additional care for pregnancy complications, since up to half of those initially categorized as 'low risk' will develop complications during their pregnancy, often of a minor and transient nature requiring only a small degree of medical input under a shared-care philosophy.

Over the last two decades several government working documents have recommended an integrated model of antenatal care aimed at improving continuity, minimizing duplication of effort by reducing the number of antenatal visits, and improving care quality by integrating antenatal education and clinical care in each visit.[1]

Basic principles of antenatal care

The principles that should underpin antenatal care have been summarized in a guidance document published by NICE.[6] They are as follows:

- Midwives and GPs should care for women with an uncomplicated pregnancy, providing continuous care throughout the pregnancy. Obstetricians and specialist teams should be involved where additional care is needed.
- Antenatal appointments should take place in a location that women can easily access. The location should be appropriate to the needs of the woman and her community.
- Maternity records should be national, structured and standardized, and held by the woman.
- In an uncomplicated pregnancy, there should be 10 appointments for nulliparous women and 7 for parous women.
- Each antenatal appointment should have a structure and a focus. Appointments early in pregnancy should be longer, to provide information and time for discussion about screening so that the woman can make informed decisions.
- If possible, routine tests should be incorporated into the appointments to minimize inconvenience to women.
- Women should feel able to discuss sensitive issues and disclose problems. Practitioners should be alert to the symptoms and signs of domestic violence and abuse.

Organization and content of the antenatal visit

It is increasingly recognized that the content of an antenatal visit consultation should be well defined and streamlined, incorporating a combination of clinical assessments and screening tests for which evidence of clinical benefit has been scientifically evaluated. Broadly, the evaluation should incorporate those assessments and tests that seek to identify existing or emerging risks for the mother and the unborn child. Clarification needs to be provided regarding the first point of contact of the pregnant woman with her care professional. Guidelines for care should detail the essential requirements of the booking visit and the core needs for a follow-up consultation visit. To take full advantage of antenatal care, women should ideally book in the first trimester, as it is well recognized that 'late bookers' are at increased risk of adverse pregnancy outcomes. Following the first visit, the frequency and content of subsequent antenatal visits should be explained clearly and simply so that women and all caregivers understand what is required.

FREQUENCY OF ANTENATAL VISITS

The optimum number of antenatal care clinic visits has been the subject of intense discussion. Since the 1920s, when a national system of antenatal clinics with a uniform pattern of visits and procedures was introduced in the UK, the average number of visits has reduced from up to 14 to as low as 8, with no associated adverse effects in clinical outcome.

In developed countries with well-established maternity services, small reductions in the number of antenatal visits are compatible with good perinatal outcomes. One study in London found that women with more frequent antenatal visits did not demonstrate any clinical benefit but were more likely to be satisfied with their overall care.[7] Data from developing countries is not as clear-cut, but one trial conducted in Zimbabwe suggested that modest reductions in numbers of clinic visits may not adversely affect clinical outcomes in particular settings where the quality of care provided during each visit is good.[8] Taken together, flexible individualized approaches to the provision of psychosocial support and care need not necessitate frequent hospital visits.

A care structure that enables women to contact their care provider by telephone may minimize the need for clinic visits without reducing the quality of care provided. These observations have informed NICE guidance, which stipulates that nulliparous woman with an uncomplicated pregnancy should have about 10 clinic appointments, while a schedule of 7 appointments should suffice for a woman who is parous with an uncomplicated pregnancy.[6] Clearly women who have identified risk factors for adverse pregnancy outcome may benefit from more frequent visits and investigations.

There is often a distinction made between the first contact of the pregnant woman with a health professional and the formal booking visit. It is often the case that the first contact is with the woman's GP or a designated midwife, either at the GP surgery or, more commonly, at the woman's home.

FIRST CONTACT WITH A HEALTHCARE PROFESSIONAL

This should occur soon after pregnancy has been confirmed. It provides an opportunity to obtain clinical information about the woman, provide her with information about pregnancy, and establish basic care pathways. Specific information should be given on:

- folic acid supplements
- food hygiene, including how to reduce the risk of a food-acquired infection
- lifestyle, including smoking cessation, recreational drug use and alcohol consumption
- antenatal screening, including risks, benefits and limitations of the screening tests

THE BOOKING VISIT

This should happen ideally between 8 and 12 weeks gestation and should aim to identify women who may need additional care, and to plan the pattern of care for the pregnancy. It should include the following checks and tests:

- Measure height and weight and calculate body mass index (BMI).
- Measure blood pressure and test urine for proteinuria.
- Determine risk factors for pre-eclampsia and gestational diabetes.
- Offer blood tests to check blood group and rhesus D status, and screen for anaemia, haemoglobinopathies, red-cell alloantibodies, hepatitis B virus, HIV, rubella susceptibility and syphilis.
- Offer screening for asymptomatic bacteriuria.
- Inform women younger than 25 years about the high prevalence of chlamydia infection in their age group, and provide details of their local screening or testing service.
- Offer screening for Down's syndrome. In the UK, screening for Edwards' syndrome and Patau's syndrome is now also routinely offered in the first trimester.[9]
- Offer early ultrasound scan for gestational age assessment, and ultrasound screening for structural anomalies.
- Identify women who have had genital mutilation.
- Ask about any past or present severe mental illness or psychiatric treatment.
- Ask about mood, to identify possible depression.
- Ask about the woman's occupation, to identify potential risks.

Specific information should be given, both verbally and through specially designed information, on:
- how the baby develops during pregnancy
- nutrition and diet, including vitamin D supplements
- exercise, including pelvic floor exercises
- antenatal screening, including risks and benefits of the screening tests
- the pregnancy care pathway
- planning place of birth
- breastfeeding, including workshops
- participant-led antenatal classes
- maternity benefits

FOLLOW-UP VISITS

- A visit at 16 weeks provides an opportunity to review, discuss and record the results of screening tests performed earlier, measure blood pressure and test urine for proteinuria, and offer additional investigations and iron supplementation if the maternal haemoglobin level is below 11 g/dL. Specific information regarding the routine anomaly scan should also be provided and the scan should be offered.
- If the woman elects to have an anomaly ultrasound scan to screen for structural anomalies, this should be performed between 18 and 21 weeks. For a woman

whose placenta extends across the internal cervical os, another scan should be offered at 32 weeks to exclude placenta praevia.

- At 28 weeks gestation all women should be seen for additional checks and tests. Blood pressure should be measured and the urine tested for proteinuria. Women should be offered a second screening test for anaemia and atypical red-cell alloantibodies. A haemoglobin level below 10.5 g/dL should be investigated and iron supplementation considered. Anti-D prophylaxis should be offered to women who are rhesus D (RhD) negative. Uterine size should be plotted as the symphysis–fundal height.

- For nulliparous women, a further visit at approximately 32 weeks enables documentation and discussion of the results of screening tests undertaken at 28 weeks, as well as routine measurement of blood pressure, urinalysis for proteinuria, and symphysis–fundal height assessment.

- At 34 weeks, the results of screening tests undertaken at 28 weeks should be reviewed and discussed, blood pressure and urinalysis determined, and a second dose of anti-D prophylaxis given to women who are RhD negative according to institutional guidelines. Specific information should be given regarding preparation for labour and birth, including the birth plan, recognizing active labour and coping with pain.

- In addition to routine assessments, the finding of breech presentation at 36 weeks should mandate a discussion of external cephalic version. Advice regarding breastfeeding, care of the new baby, vitamin K prophylaxis and newborn screening tests, as well as an awareness of the features of postnatal depression, should be offered. It is customary to arrange elective indicated abdominal delivery at 36 weeks for a date and time that would depend on the indication for such operative delivery.

- Subsequent antenatal visits should happen at 38, 40 and 41 weeks. These should include routine assessments with additional emphasis aimed at planning for the imminent birth of the baby. Particular attention should be paid at these visits to fetal size and presentation, and emphasis should be placed on deciding the timing of the delivery. If spontaneous labour is planned, a decision regarding the timing of labour initiation should be made at one of these later visits, depending on the presence of any risk factors for late fetal demise or maternal medical deterioration. For women who have not given birth by 41 weeks, a membrane sweep should also be offered. Induction of labour should also be discussed and offered

GENERAL LIFESTYLE ADVICE DURING PREGNANCY

During the course of pregnancy, care providers should make every effort to provide relevant advice and support to pregnant women regarding lifestyle issues and habits about which they may feel ignorant. While there is a dearth of evidence regarding the risks of some lifestyle issues and practices during pregnancy, the safety and impact of many are well established. Advice should therefore routinely cover these lifestyle issues, as well as educating women about practices which are best avoided and those which promote good health during pregnancy. Table 1.1 summarizes the common areas such as work, sex, nutrition, exercise and the intake of food supplements about which advice should be given during antenatal care.

Table 1.1 Advice during antenatal care regarding risks associated with lifestyle choices (adapted from NICE Clinical Guideline 62, *Antenatal Care: Routine Care for the Healthy Pregnant Woman*[6])

Complementary therapies	Few complementary therapies have been proven to be safe and effective during pregnancy.
Exercise	No risk associated with moderate exercise. Avoid sports that may cause abdominal trauma, falls and excessive joint stress.
Sexual intercourse	Intercourse thought to be safe during uncomplicated pregnancy.
Alcohol	The safest approach is not to drink alcohol at all when pregnant or planning a pregnancy.[10] If women choose to drink, drink no more than 1–2 UK units once or twice a week (1 unit equals half a pint of ordinary-strength lager or beer, or one shot [25 mL] of spirits. One small [125 mL] glass of wine is equal to 1.5 UK units). Advise women to avoid getting drunk and to avoid binge drinking.
Smoking	Discuss smoking status and give information about risks during pregnancy. Give information, advice and support to stop smoking during pregnancy. Refer to appropriate stop-smoking services and pregnancy smoking helplines. Discuss nicotine replacement therapy (NRT).
Work	Usually safe to continue working for most occupations. Refer to the Health and Safety Executive for more information. Inform about maternity rights and benefits.
Nutritional supplements	Recommend supplementation with folic acid before conception and throughout the first 12 weeks (400 μg per day). Advise of importance of vitamin D intake during pregnancy and breastfeeding (10 μg per day). Ensure women at risk of deficiency are following this advice. Routine iron supplementation not recommended. Advise of risk of birth defects with vitamin A, and to avoid vitamin A supplementation and liver products.
Avoiding infection	Advise how to reduce the risk of listeriosis and salmonella, and how to avoid toxoplasmosis infection.
Medicines	Prescribe as few medicines as possible, and only in circumstances where the benefit outweighs the risk. Advise avoidance of over-the-counter medicines.
Cannabis	Discourage women from using cannabis.
Air travel	Long-haul air travel is associated with an increased risk of venous thrombosis. Advise compression stockings to reduce the risk.
Car travel	Seatbelt should go 'above and below the bump, not over it'.
Travel abroad	Advise women to discuss flying, vaccinations and travel insurance with their midwife or doctor.

PRE-PREGNANCY COUNSELLING AND CARE

For women with specific problems, such as a history of fetal abnormality or a medical condition such as epilepsy or thrombophilia, pre-pregnancy care is required. Many of the factors operating to associate such conditions with adverse obstetric outcome can only be addressed adequately before pregnancy. Such care will not only prevent or modify the risk of adverse outcome, but will also allow the woman to make an informed choice as to whether to proceed with a pregnancy, to time it optimally, and to obtain appropriate information and advice on the management of any pregnancy. Choices made at this time are preferable to difficult decisions when problems are encountered antenatally.

Key summary points

- Antenatal care is crucial for optimizing pregnancy outcomes for both high-risk and low-risk pregnancies.

- Identification and management of risk is a cardinal aim of antenatal care.

- Early first attendance for care is associated with better pregnancy outcomes than late booking and poor engagement in regular care.

- The midwife and GP should provide the majority of care for women at low risk of pregnancy complications, while a consultant obstetrician should provide major input into the care for women with medical, social or gestational risks. It may be necessary to organize services such that specialist clinics have an input into the care of women with medical or obstetric complications.

- Pre-pregnancy care and counselling should be readily accessible to all women of childbearing age to enable careful planning so that women become pregnant in the best possible health. Such care should include ready access to appropriate contraception.

References

1. Department of Health. *Changing Childbirth: Report of the Expert Maternity Group*. London: HMSO, 1993.

2. Department of Health. *Maternity Matters: Choice, Access and Continuity of Care in a Safe Service*. London: HMSO, 2007.

3. Alexander S, Keirse MJNC. Formal risk scoring in pregnancy. In Chalmers I, Enkin M, Keirse MJNC, eds. *Effective Care in Pregnancy and Childbirth*. Oxford: Oxford University Press, 1989, pp. 345–65.

4. Cole S, McIlwaine G. The use of risk factors in predicting possible consequences of changing patterns of care in pregnancy. In Chamberlain G, Patel N, eds. *The Future of Maternity Services*. London: RCOG Press, 1994, pp. 65–72.

5. Tucker JS, Hall MH, Howie PW, *et al.* Should obstetricians see women with normal pregnancies? A multicentre randomised controlled trial of routine antenatal care by general practitioners and midwives compared with shared care led by obstetricians. *BMJ* 1996; 312: 554–9.

6. National Institute for Health and Care Excellence (NICE). *Antenatal Care: Routine Care for the Healthy Pregnant Woman*. NICE Clinical Guideline CG62. London: NICE, 2008.

7. Sikorski J, Wilson J, Clement S, *et al*. A randomised controlled trial comparing two schedules of antenatal visits: the antenatal care project. *BMJ* 1996; 312: 546–53.

8. Munjanja SP, Lindmark G, Nystrom L. Randomised controlled trial of a reduced-visits programme of antenatal care in Harare, Zimbabwe. *Lancet* 1996; 348: 364–9.

9. Public Health England. *Screening Tests for You and Your Baby*. London: Department of Health, 2014. www.gov.uk/topic/population-screening-programmes (accessed 3 April 2016).

10. Department of Health. *UK Chief Medical Officers' Alcohol Guidelines Review: Summary of the Proposed New Guidelines*. London: Department of Health, 2015.

2 Antepartum haemorrhage

Hannah Yeeles and Swati Jha

Introduction

Antepartum haemorrhage (APH) is defined as any bleeding from or into the genital tract from 24 weeks gestation until the birth of the baby. It complicates 3–5% of pregnancies and is a leading cause of perinatal and maternal morbidity and mortality worldwide. The most significant causes of APH are placental abruption and placenta praevia (Table 2.1). However, more commonly, bleeding occurs secondary to local and unexplained causes.

There are no consistent classifications for the severity of APH. The following definitions are widely used:[1]

- *Spotting* – staining, streaking or blood spotting noted on underwear or sanitary protection
- *Minor haemorrhage* – blood loss < 50 mL that has settled
- *Major haemorrhage* – blood loss of 50–1000 mL, with no signs of shock
- *Massive haemorrhage* – blood loss greater than 1000 mL and/or signs of clinical shock

The amount of blood loss is frequently underestimated. The mother's general condition, and in particular signs of shock, can help to determine the severity of the bleeding. Fetal distress or demise is a good indicator of significant volume depletion.

General management principles

The basic principles of resuscitation should be followed in a woman presenting with major APH or collapse. This should include a primary survey with a structured approach for checking the airways, breathing and circulation ('ABC'). Following this, causes should be considered and specific management tailored to this.

Antenatal Disorders for the MRCOG and Beyond, Second Edition, ed. Dilly Anumba and Shehnaaz Jivraj. Published by Cambridge University Press. © Cambridge University Press 2016.

Table 2.1 Summary of causes of APH

Obstetric	Non-obstetric	Other bleeding (not from vagina)
Bloody show	Cervical bleeding	GI bleeding
Placental abruption	• ectropion	• haemorrhoids
Placenta praevia	• cervicitis	• inflammatory bowel
Vasa praevia	• polyp	Urinary tract
Marginal bleed	• neoplasm	• infection
Uterine rupture	Vaginal bleeding	
	• trauma	
	• neoplasm	

Abdominal palpation should be performed. A soft, non-tender uterus may suggest placenta praevia or local causes. On the other hand, a tender hard uterus would be more in keeping with placental abruption. Speculum examination is helpful to assess for vaginal or cervical causes and may reveal cervical dilatation. Digital vaginal examination should *not* be performed until placenta praevia has been excluded.

All RhD-negative women should have a Kleihauer test performed to quantify fetomaternal haemorrhage. Anti-D immunoglobulin must be given to all non-sensitized RhD-negative women after any presentation of APH. In minor haemorrhage, a full blood count (FBC) and group and save should be requested. In major APH, in addition to FBC, blood should be obtained for clotting screen, renal and liver function, and four units of red cells crossmatched. Clotting factors including platelets, fresh frozen plasma (FFP) and cryoprecipitate are likely to be required if more than 4–6 units of blood are transfused.

Once resuscitation has commenced and/or the mother is stable, fetal assessment with a cardiotocograph (CTG) should be performed. This may influence the timing and mode of delivery. If the fetal heart cannot be auscultated, an ultrasound scan is indicated to exclude an intrauterine fetal death.

If there is maternal and/or fetal compromise, an obstetric emergency should be declared. Immediate delivery is recommended once resuscitation of the mother has been commenced. In situations where there is fetal distress, the priority is to stabilize the mother, while preparing to deliver the fetus. Delivery is usually by caesarean section in these circumstances, unless the woman is in established labour, there are no contraindications and vaginal delivery is imminent. If fetal death is diagnosed, vaginal birth is recommended, but caesarean section may be indicated in some cases.

Placental abruption

Placental abruption is the premature separation of a normally implanted placenta from the uterine wall, resulting in haemorrhage before the delivery of the fetus. In severe cases, it is associated with significant perinatal morbidity and mortality. The severity of fetal distress correlates with the degree of placental separation. In near-complete or complete abruption, fetal death is inevitable, unless there is immediate delivery. Although maternal mortality is rare, morbidity can result from haemorrhage, shock, disseminated intravascular coagulation (DIC) and renal failure.

PATHOPHYSIOLOGY

This is usually of a normally sited placenta but can also occur in relation to a low-lying placenta. Abruption arises from bleeding into the decidua basalis, which results in the formation of a haematoma and subsequent increase in hydrostatic pressure. This in turn leads to a separation of the adjacent placenta. In its pregnant, distended state the uterus is unable to contract around the uterine vessels at the placental site, so the bleeding persists. The expanding clot can dissect between the fetal membranes and present as vaginal bleeding or remain confined within the uterus and behind the placenta. The amount of visible bleeding is therefore a poor reflection of the actual extent of blood loss. The placental separation can be partial and self-limiting or complete, leading to the potentially devastating consequences of catastrophic bleeding and fetal demise. Damage to the fetus results from decreased placental perfusion, caused by the clot forming a barrier between the placental bed and the villi, in addition to the release of prostaglandins, which cause uterine spasm.

Occasionally, and particularly with concealed abruption, there may be bleeding into the muscles and blood vessels of the uterus, causing injury and damage. Blood can leak out of the damaged vessels and collect in the uterine muscles, causing oedema and necrosis. It is the infiltration of blood into the myometrium that is associated with pain and sustained uterine contraction, making the uterus feel 'woody' on examination. This is also responsible for provoking labour and reducing uteroplacental flow. Abruptions are painful and, in contrast to labour, the pain can be constant.

Minute bruises and ecchymoses may appear on the surface of the uterus causing it to look blotchy-blue. This is known as Couvelaire uterus, a rare but serious consequence of abruption.

AETIOLOGY

While there are several risk factors associated with placental abruption, causal pathways remain speculative. The most predictive risk is abruption in a previous pregnancy. The recurrence rate in subsequent pregnancies is 7–9%, which increases to 19–25% in those women who have had two previous pregnancies complicated by abruption.

First-trimester bleeding increases the risk of abruption later in the pregnancy. Women with ultrasound-detected subchorionic haemorrhage before 22 weeks of gestation have been found to be at increased risk of placental abruption and

Table 2.2 Risk factors associated with placental abruption

Maternal	Obstetric/fetal	Other
Previous abruption	Fetal growth restriction	Abdominal trauma
Advanced maternal age	Polyhydramnios	
Multiparity	Pre-eclampsia	
Low body mass index (BMI)	Non-vertex presentations	
Smoking and drug misuse (tobacco, cocaine and amphetamines)	Intrauterine infection	
Hypertension	Premature rupture of membranes	

preterm delivery but are not at increased risk of other adverse pregnancy outcomes.[2]

Some disorders characterized by thrombophilia have also been implicated in the past, particularly factor V Leiden and prothrombin gene mutation; however, the association is weak.

In view of the known links with tobacco, cocaine and amphetamines, women should be encouraged to abstain from these. Table 2.2 summarizes the risk factors for placental abruption.

CLINICAL PRESENTATION

The diagnosis of abruption is made on the basis of clinical presentation. Ultrasound imaging of the placenta is of limited diagnostic value except in cases of large retroplacental haematoma, where the positive predictive value is high. In severe cases, there may be heavy vaginal bleeding and acute abdominal pain. Serous fluid from a retroplacental haematoma may trickle out and be confused with amniotic fluid. 50% of patients will present in labour, and rupturing the membranes may demonstrate blood-stained liquor. Classically, the uterus is tender and tense, often described as 'woody hard'. There may be uterine irritability and palpable contractions or hypertonus, resulting in labour. Fetal distress or intrauterine fetal death may be diagnosed. The woman may be in hypovolaemic shock. However, sometimes the diagnosis of abruption is not so obvious, particularly when the symptoms and signs are more subtle.

Broadly speaking, there are three types of placental abruption:

- *Revealed* – The bleeding flows down between the membranes and the uterine wall and is revealed at the introitus. Since there is little or no collection of blood behind the placenta, separation from the uterus is usually less than in the other types.
- *Concealed* – The blood collects between the placenta and the uterine wall and fails to trickle out of the vagina. The extent of bleeding is therefore frequently underestimated. Blood clot can continue to dissect the placenta from its uterine

Table 2.3 Clinical classification of placental abruption based on severity[3]

Class	Incidence	Features/characteristics
Class 0 – asymptomatic		Made retrospectively by finding an organized clot or depressed area in the placenta
Class 1 – mild	48%	No/minimal vaginal bleeding
		No maternal or fetal compromise
Class 2 – moderate	27%	No/moderate vaginal bleeding
		Moderate uterine tenderness
		Maternal tachycardia, orthostatic changes in BP and heart rate
		Fetal distress
Class 3 – severe	24%	No/heavy vaginal bleeding
		Very painful hypertonic contractions
		Maternal shock
		Coagulopathy
		Fetal death

bed and separate over large areas, sometime completely. This is typically the severe type of abruption.

- *Mixed* – This presents with bleeding but there is also concealed bleeding behind the placenta. This should be suspected when the degree of compromise is out of proportion to the bleeding.

The severity of placental abruption can be classified based on various clinical features. This is shown in Table 2.3.

MANAGEMENT

In mild placental abruption, the bleeding may settle and the symptoms gradually resolve. With satisfactory fetal monitoring these women can often be managed as outpatients. It is not always possible to distinguish between idiopathic preterm labour and mild abruption, and thus these women should have continuous electronic fetal monitoring and careful observation.

The management goals in moderate or severe placental abruption are to correct the hypovolaemia, deliver the fetus and observe for and correct any coagulation defect that arises. This requires management in the labour ward, with intensive monitoring of both mother and fetus.

The management of severe abruption requires a multidisciplinary team approach, and the protocol for massive APH should be implemented. Initial management should follow the ABC pathway for resuscitation. Two large-bore intravenous lines are required and blood should be sent urgently, including a crossmatch of four units. An indwelling catheter should be inserted. As the woman is being stabilized, the fetus can be assessed and a plan made for delivery.

Resuscitation and caesarean section/induction of labour can happen simultaneously, and in the event of fetal distress delivery should be undertaken without delay. Placental abruption often precipitates rapid labour, and vaginal delivery may be possible in the absence of fetal distress. Artificial rupture of the membranes should be performed to expedite labour.

The aim of resuscitation is to achieve safe delivery of the fetus and to enter the third stage of labour with a normal blood pressure (BP), central venous pressure (CVP) and urine output, and corrected DIC.

As per Royal College of Obstetricians and Gynaecologists (RCOG) guidance, there are four pillars of management:

1. communication between all members of the multidisciplinary team
2. resuscitation
3. monitoring and investigation
4. arresting bleeding by arranging delivery of the fetus

After delivery of the fetus, there is a significant risk of postpartum haemorrhage. This can be particularly serious, since the patient may already be compromised with an impaired ability to withstand further blood loss.

Following a massive APH, regardless of the outcome, it is essential that an experienced obstetrician debrief the woman and her partner regarding the course of events. Access for medical and psychological support should be made readily available.

Fluid management of hypovolaemia

The priority is to restore effective circulating volume to optimize tissue perfusion. This can be achieved with crystalloid or colloid solutions until blood and plasma are available. The crystalloid solutions that may be given include normal saline or Hartmann's solution, but non-salt crystalloids such as 5% dextrose are ineffective. Care should be taken when using colloids in the event of fluid overload and/or pulmonary oedema. Fluid replacement volumes should be two or three times the estimated blood loss to account for fluid shifts into the extravascular compartments. The response to fluid resuscitation can be monitored using CVP and urine output (> 0.5 mg/kg/hour).

Coagulopathy/disseminated intravascular coagulation (DIC)

Coagulation failure can progress rapidly or take hours to evolve. This is more common in severe abruption and is associated with fetal death. The diagnosis of DIC is by a combination of the clinical presentation and laboratory test results as shown in Table 2.4. The degree of the coagulation disorder depends on the amount of blood loss and the release of pro-coagulant substances (thromboplastins from placental injury) into the maternal circulation. There is an endothelial response

Table 2.4   The laboratory features of coagulopathy in abruption

Activated partial thromboplastin time prolonged

Prothrombin time prolonged

Thrombin time prolonged

Fibrinogen low for pregnancy, though it may still be within normal limits

Platelets low

Fibrin degradation products increased

caused by tissue hypoxia and hypovolaemia, which leads to production of oxygen free radicals and pro-inflammatory cytokines. Endothelial damage and thrombo-plastins result in widespread activation of the clotting cascade. There is increased vascular permeability and loss of vascular integrity. Rapid consumption of platelets and coagulation factors ensues, with defibrination, thrombocytopenia and overall failure of haemostasis.

The management of DIC involves treating the underlying cause, i.e. delivering the fetus and placenta, in addition to replacing and maintaining blood and clotting products. Fibrinogen is the pro-coagulant that is most often required, and this is replaced in the form of fresh frozen plasma (FFP).

Placenta praevia

Placenta praevia exists when the placenta is inserted partially or wholly into the lower segment of the uterus. Maternal and fetal morbidity and mortality are considerable. Symptomatic placenta praevia affects between 0.4% and 0.8% of pregnancies.

It is classified by ultrasound imaging (Table 2.5); if the placenta is covering the cervical os it is considered a major placenta praevia (types III and IV). If the leading edge of the placenta is in the lower segment but not covering the cervical os, a minor or partial praevia exists (types I and II) (Figure 2.1). Grading the placenta praevia is very important in order to determine the correct management.

Table 2.5   The classification of placenta praevia based on ultrasound scan findings

Type	Description
Type I	The placenta encroaches into the lower uterine segment and lies within 5 cm of the internal cervical os
Type II	The placenta reaches the cervical os but does not cover it
Type III	The placenta covers the cervical os but the placental site is asymmetric with most of the placenta being on one side of the cervical os
Type IV	The placenta is centrally located over the cervical os

Table 2.6 Risk factors for placenta praevia

Previous placenta praevia

Previous caesarean section(s)

Previous termination of pregnancy

Multiparity

Advanced maternal age (> 40 years)

Multiple pregnancy

Smoking

Assisted conception

Deficient endometrium due to presence or history of:

– uterine scar

– endometritis

– manual removal of placenta

– curettage

– submucous fibroid

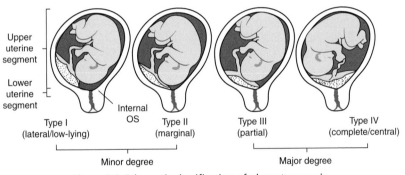

Figure 2.1 Schematic classification of placenta praevia.

AETIOLOGY AND RISK FACTORS

The exact aetiology of placenta praevia is unknown, but it is likely to be related to conditions existing prior to pregnancy. A number of risk factors have been identified, as shown in Table 2.6. A possible hypothesis is that placenta praevia is related to abnormal vascularization of the endometrium caused by scarring or atrophy from previous trauma, surgery or infection.

DIAGNOSIS

The diagnosis of placenta praevia is made by ultrasound. Up to 26% of placentas are found to be low-lying at the routine anatomy scan at about 20 weeks gestation. However, during the late second and third trimester there is placental migration as the lower segment develops. Only 5% of placentas remain low-lying at 32 weeks gestation. In asymptomatic cases of minor placenta praevia, follow-up ultrasound evaluation should be performed at 36 weeks gestation. In women with asymptomatic major praevia, further scanning should be performed at 32 weeks to allow time for planning for further imaging and delivery. If the placenta is still low-lying at this stage, the majority (73%) will remain so at term, although in cases of major praevia 90% persist.

In women who have had a previous caesarean section there are two potential problems: placenta praevia and placenta accreta. If the placenta is anterior and reaches the os, further imaging is advised to determine whether it has implanted into the caesarean section scar. Transvaginal scanning and magnetic resonance imaging may help to facilitate the diagnosis.

CLINICAL PRESENTATION

Classical placenta praevia presents with varying degrees of painless vaginal bleeding. The loss is usually bright red because it remains oxygenated (in contrast to placental abruption, which is darker in colour). The bleeding may have been provoked by sexual intercourse or the onset of labour.

The woman may be in shock, depending on the amount of bleeding. The uterus is usually soft and non-tender, and if there are contractions palpable, the uterus will relax in between. Speculum examination may be helpful to determine the amount of bleeding and exclude other causes. Digital vaginal examination is contraindicated, particularly in cases where the placental site is unknown.

Clinical suspicion should be high in all women with vaginal bleeding after 20 weeks gestation. A high presenting part, abnormal lie and painless or provoked vaginal bleeding, irrespective of previous imaging, should raise the question of a low-lying placenta.

MANAGEMENT

There remains a lack of evidence to guide place of care (hospital versus home), and management should be tailored to the individual's needs. No significant differences in maternal or fetal outcome have been reported for women staying at home, compared with those kept in hospital. Previous guidance suggested admitting women at 34 weeks gestation with major placenta praevia who have previously bled. Currently, this will vary between obstetric units and should be judged on a case-by-case basis.

Women with a low-lying placenta in the third trimester should be counselled about the risk of haemorrhage and preterm delivery. They should be encouraged to attend immediately in the event of bleeding, any abdominal pain or tightenings. In cases of home-based care, there should be rapid access to hospital and someone available to assist them at all times. The clinical course of placenta praevia is difficult to predict, and women may require several admissions to hospital with recurrent bleeding episodes. A Kleihauer test should be performed with every episode of bleeding in rhesus-negative women, and anti-D immunoglobulin administered as required. Monitoring and treatment for anaemia should be aggressive, given the significant risk of antepartum and postpartum haemorrhage.

DELIVERY

The mode of delivery should be based on clinical judgement and guided by ultrasound findings. The woman's preferences should also be taken into consideration, particularly if the fetal head has entered the pelvis.

Caesarean section is the usual mode of delivery for grade III and IV placenta praevias, and most grade II. If the placental edge is less than 2 cm from the internal os in the third trimester, delivery by caesarean section is likely. However, the lower uterine segment will continue to develop, and further imaging with transvaginal scanning may be helpful in those women planning a caesarean section where the fetal head is engaged.

Elective delivery by caesarean section in women who are asymptomatic should be performed after 38 weeks gestation. If placenta accreta is suspected, delivery is advised at 36–37 weeks. Delivery should be in a unit with blood bank facilities and high-dependency care because of the risk of major haemorrhage and hysterectomy. Sequential reports of the Confidential Enquiries into Maternal Deaths in the UK have recommended that the operator at a caesarean section for placenta praevia should be senior (consultant or senior registrar grade).[4] A consultant anaesthetist should also be present.

In an acute situation, the degree of bleeding may be variable and cannot be predicted from the grade of placenta praevia. Management depends on the degree of haemorrhage and fetal maturity. Indications for delivery before 37 weeks gestation include:

- onset of labour
- fetal distress
- severe bleeding which is life-threatening to the mother
- intrauterine death

Blood should be available promptly during the peripartum period. The need to crossmatch blood will depend on the clinical situation and local blood bank policies. Specific plans will need to be in place for those women with atypical antibodies. Cell salvage can be used, and is particularly important in women who decline blood products.

Vasa praevia

Vasa praevia describes fetal blood vessels running through the membranes over the internal cervical os and below the presenting part, unprotected by placental tissue. This can be:

- vasa praevia type 1 – secondary to a velamentous cord insertion in a single or bilobed placenta
- vasa praevia type 2 – from the fetal vessels running between lobes of placenta with one or more accessory lobes

Maternal size, the status of the maternal bladder, and the orientation of vessels as they cross the lower uterine segment may limit visualization of the offending fetal vessels.

CLINICAL PRESENTATION

These fetal blood vessels are at risk of rupture when the supporting membranes rupture, posing significant risk to the fetus. Vasa praevia may present with vaginal bleeding at the time of rupture of membranes associated with fetal heart rate abnormalities including decelerations, bradycardia and, at worst, fetal demise. Uncommonly, bleeding can occur in the absence of ruptured membranes. The loss of small amounts of blood can have major implications for the fetus, owing to the relatively low fetal circulating volume (80–100 mL/kg). Prompt delivery and transfusion of blood, if required, is essential.

RISK FACTORS

These include conditions associated with vessels that run close to the cervix: low-lying placenta, placenta praevia, multiple pregnancies, in-vitro fertilization, and multiloculate and velamentous cord insertion.

DIAGNOSIS

Vasa praevia is unlikely to present as an *antepartum* haemorrhage. The usual diagnosis is on vaginal examination with palpation of fetal vessels, vaginal bleeding after an artificial rupture of the membranes or a pathological trace in labour, particularly sinusoidal patterns. Vasa praevia can be recognized on grey-scale ultrasound scan as linear structures in front of the internal os. Arterial and venous flow can be identified by Doppler studies. A transvaginal scan is superior to an abdominal scan.

MANAGEMENT AND PROGNOSIS

The major complication from vasa praevia is rupture of the vessels carrying fetal blood, leading to fetal anaemia. A rare complication is fetal hypoxia, caused by compression of the fetal blood vessels by the presenting part. It is associated with significant perinatal mortality in undiagnosed cases.

When detected antenatally, delivery is safest by caesarean section prior to the onset of labour. The optimal gestational age at delivery has not been established; it is usually recommended that delivery happens by 35–36 weeks,[5] but individualized care is necessary. The outcome is greatly improved (up to 97%) when a prenatal diagnosis is made. It would be reasonable to consider hospital admission from 30–32 weeks gestation, in addition to administration of corticosteroids for promotion of lung maturity.

Marginal bleed

The presentation of marginal bleeding is similar to a placenta praevia, but it occurs from the edge of a normally situated placenta after 28 weeks gestation. Marginal haemorrhages occur because of contraction of the lower uterine segment beneath the lower pole of the placenta. This may lead to vaginal bleeding, but cases demonstrate no pathological lesion, no fetal compromise, and no association with maternal disease. It is important to distinguish marginal bleeding from vasa praevia.

In other cases, the dissection of a retroplacental haematoma to the lower margin of the placenta may permit vaginal bleeding, decompressing the haematoma and perhaps preventing a more complete separation of the placenta. An alternative theory of marginal haemorrhage is the rupture of the large veins at the periphery of the placenta in the decidua and myometrium.

The general condition of the patient is proportionate to the amount of bleeding, as all the blood loss is revealed.

Management is dependent on the overall condition of the woman, the gestation, and whether she is in labour. If labour is confirmed, vaginal delivery should be expedited by amniotomy and oxytocin infusion. For patients not in labour with severe bleeding, a caesarean section may be required. If the bleeding is slight, but gestational age is more than 37 weeks, induction of labour is indicated. If gestational age is less than 37 weeks, the patient is usually managed conservatively.

Uterine rupture

Uterine rupture is a rare and catastrophic complication of pregnancy with a high maternal and fetal morbidity and mortality rate. It can occur in women with an unscarred uterus, or a uterus with a previous surgical scar. There is full-thickness disruption of the uterine wall, which also involves the visceral peritoneum. It is associated with clinically significant uterine bleeding, fetal distress and expulsion of the fetus/and or placenta into the abdominal cavity.

RISK FACTORS

Several factors increase the risk of uterine rupture. These include congenital uterine abnormalities, uterine trauma, previous uterine myomectomy, the number and type of previous caesarean section deliveries, grand multiparity, induction of labour, and fetal macrosomia.

CLINICAL PRESENTATION

The symptoms and signs of uterine rupture depend on the site, time and extent of the defect. Classically, there is:

- fetal distress (decelerations, bradycardia)
- loss of uterine contractility
- abdominal pain
- recession of the presenting part
- haemorrhage
- shock

However, it has been shown that some of these features are rare and not reliably distinguished from other obstetric complications.

MANAGEMENT

The most important initial management is to establish the diagnosis in a timely manner. It is then imperative to stabilize the mother and deliver the fetus. After delivery, the type of surgical treatment for the mother will depend on the type and extent of rupture, the degree of bleeding and the desire for future pregnancies. Hysterectomy may be preferred when there is intractable bleeding or when the uterine rupture sites are multiple, low-lying or longitudinal.

Unexplained bleeding

Unexplained bleeding is a common diagnosis for women presenting with APH. Women usually complain of painless vaginal bleeding, which may be provoked or unprovoked. Pregnancies complicated by unexplained bleeding are also at risk of adverse perinatal outcomes. A recent study found that these women are at greater risk of preterm delivery and undergoing induction of labour, and their babies are more likely to be admitted to the neonatal unit.

Other causes of bleeding of unexplained/uncertain origin include:

- cervical lesions (e.g. cervical polyp or ectropion, which may cause bleeding, but usually only postcoitally)
- vaginal lesions
- excessive show
- rectal bleeding mistaken for vaginal (e.g. haemorrhoids or fissures)

MANAGEMENT

This should include a detailed history and examination. Speculum examination may reveal a vaginal or cervical cause. A woman with a clinically suspicious cervix should be referred for colposcopic evaluation. Swabs may be indicated if infection is suspected. An ultrasound scan should be performed to exclude placenta praevia.

Women who present with spotting that has settled may be reassured and sent home. All women with heavier than spotting or ongoing bleeding should be offered admission and observed until it has resolved. The optimal time for delivery in women with unexplained bleeding is not established and needs to be determined by a senior obstetrician.

Key summary points

- Antepartum haemorrhage (APH) is a leading cause of perinatal and maternal morbidity and mortality worldwide.

- A high presenting part, abnormal lie and painless or provoked vaginal bleeding, irrespective of previous imaging, should raise the question of a low-lying placenta.

- A multidisciplinary team approach should be used for the management of massive APH. Initial management should follow the ABC pathway for resuscitation.

- Prompt management of hypovolaemia and coagulopathy is vital.

- Do not forget the patient and her partner – a debriefing of events is essential.

References

1. Royal College of Obstetricians and Gynaecologists. *Antepartum Haemorrhage*. Green-top Guideline No. 63. London: RCOG, 2011.

2. Norman SM, Odibo AO, Macones GA, *et al.* Ultrasound-detected subchorionic hemorrhage and the obstetric implications. *Obstet Gynecol* 2010; 116: 311–15.

3. Deering S. Abruptio placentae. *Medscape* 2011. http://emedicine.medscape.com/article/252810-overview (accessed 24 April 2015).

4. Knight M, Kenyon S, Brocklehurst P, *et al.*, on behalf of MBRRACEUK. *Saving Lives, Improving Mothers' Care: Lessons learned to inform future maternity care from the UK and Ireland Confidential Enquiries into Maternal Deaths and Morbidity 2009–12*. Oxford: National Perinatal Epidemiology Unit, University of Oxford, 2014.

5. Gagnon R, Morin L, Bly S, *et al.* SOGC clinical practice guideline: guidelines for the management of vasa previa. *Int J Gynaecol Obstet* 2010; 108: 85–9.

Further reading

Hall D. Abruptio placentae and disseminated intravascular coagulopathy. *Semin Perinatol* 2009; 33: 189–95.

Hall MH, Wagaarachchi P. Antepartum haemorrhage. In Maclean AB, Neilson JP, eds. *Maternal Morbidity and Mortality*. London: RCOG Press, 2002, pp. 227–40.

Royal College of Obstetricians and Gynaecologists. *Antepartum Haemorrhage*. Green-top Guideline No. 63. London: RCOG, 2011.

Royal College of Obstetricians and Gynaecologists. *Placenta Praevia, Placenta Praevia Accreta and Vasa Praevia: Diagnosis and Management*. Green-top Guideline No. 37. London: RCOG, 2011.

3 Multiple pregnancy

Chibuike Iruloh

Prevalence and epidemiology

The incidence of twin pregnancies in the UK is 1 in 80 spontaneous conceptions, with higher-order multiples approximately following Hellin's law. This states that the rate of n order of multiple pregnancy is $1 : 89^{n-1}$. The rate of monozygotic twinning is constant while the rate of dizygotic twinning is affected by family history, maternal age, the use of fertility drugs and treatment and geographical region, with the highest rate of 49 per 1000 maternities among the Yoruba of Nigeria.

The incidence of multiple pregnancies in the UK is increasing because of assisted reproduction technologies and increasing maternal age. About 25% of in-vitro fertilization pregnancies are multiple, compared to 1% for women who conceive naturally. In 2011 there were 16.1 multiple births per 1000 maternities, with women aged 45 and above having the highest multiple maternity rate of 99.3 per 1000. In that year, 11,330 women gave birth to twins, 172 to triplets and 3 to quadruplets or more. In 1976 there were 9.6 multiple maternities per 1000 maternities.[1]

Classification of multiple pregnancy

Twins result from the division of a zygote into two embryos or the fertilization and implantation of two different zygotes. Higher-order multiple pregnancies result from combinations of these two processes.

Zygosity refers to the number of zygotes involved in the twinning. Monozygotic twins result from the division of one zygote into two twins and are identical, having the same chromosomal composition. Dizygotic twins result from the fertilization and implantation of two eggs, resulting in non-identical twins that would have the same similarity as any other siblings. Twenty per cent of all twins are monozygotic.

Antenatal Disorders for the MRCOG and Beyond, Second Edition, ed. Dilly Anumba and Shehnaaz Jivraj. Published by Cambridge University Press. © Cambridge University Press 2016.

Chorionicity denotes the number of placentas present and whether they are shared or not. Monochorionic twins share the same placenta and are invariably monozygotic, while dichorionic twins have separate placentas and could be mono- or dizygotic. Higher-order pregnancies could all have separate placentas, such as trichorionic triplets, or there may be combinations such as dichorionic triplets with one triplet having a separate placenta with the other two monochorionic.[2]

Amnionicity refers to the number of amniotic sacs and whether these sacs are shared by the fetuses. Monochorionic twins can be either monoamniotic or diamniotic, while dichorionic twins are always diamniotic. Depending on the stage at which it divides into two embryos, a monozygotic pregnancy could be dichorionic (< 4 days after fertilization and 30%) or monochorionic (70%). Monochorionic twins could be diamnionitic (4–8 days post-fertilization), monoamniotic (8–13 days) or conjoined (> 13 days).

Complications

Maternal complications of multiple pregnancy are usually secondary to the increased placental mass, while fetal complications depend on the fetal number and the type of multiple pregnancy.

Maternal complications include morning sickness, miscarriage, hyperemesis, anaemia, discomfort, gestational diabetes, gestational hypertension, pre-eclampsia, placenta praevia, polyhydramnios, preterm delivery, antepartum haemorrhage and postpartum haemorrhage (Table 3.1).

Fetal complications include chromosomal and structural abnormalities, intra-uterine growth restriction and fetal death (Table 3.2). These complications could be selective, presenting management dilemmas for both the clinician and the patient. The risk of aneuploidy is dependent on the zygosity. In dizygotic twinning, as each twin is distinct, then the pregnancy risk is double that of a singleton pregnancy. For monozygotic twins, as they develop from the same zygote and are genetically similar, the pregnancy-specific risk of aneuploidy is the same as for

Table 3.1 Maternal complications of multiple pregnancy

Exaggerated symptoms of pregnancy, e.g. vomiting, discomfort

Hyperemesis

Miscarriage

Anaemia

Pre-eclampsia

Gestational diabetes mellitus

Placenta praevia

Polyhydramnios

Antepartum haemorrhage

Postpartum haemorrhage

Table 3.2   Fetal risks associated with multiple pregnancy

Complication	Incidence
Chromosomal abnormality	0.45%
Structural abnormality	3.5%
Growth restriction	29%
Preterm delivery (twins)	50%
Preterm delivery (triplets)	90%
Twin-to-twin transfusion syndrome (TTTS)	15%
Twin reversed arterial perfusion (TRAP) sequence	1%
Perinatal mortality rate (twins)	14.8 per 1000
Perinatal mortality rate (triplets)	51.8 per 1000

singleton pregnancies. Rarely there might be heterokaryotypic monozygotic twins with chromosomal discordance. This is usually accompanied by fetal anomalies.

Discordant fetal anomalies occur in 85% of anomalous twin pregnancies. While concordant anomalies are rare in dichorionic pregnancies, they occur in 18% of anomalous monochorionic pregnancies.[3] Management options are expectant care, selective feticide or termination of the entire pregnancy. Selective feticide could be performed because of the abnormality but may also be indicated for obstetric reasons to prevent such complications as pre-eclampsia, polyhydramnios and preterm delivery. These complications may result from such anomalies as anencephaly and lethal trisomies. Spontaneous death of an anomalous twin can result in the death of, or neurological injury to, the normal twin in a monochorionic pregnancy. In monochorionic twins, selective feticide must be preceded or performed by procedures that separate both fetal circulations in order to avoid risks to the surviving twin. These risks are discussed later under *Monofetal death*.

The risk of perinatal mortality is 3–6 times higher for twins (14.8 per 1000 live births) and about 9 times higher for triplets (51.8) when compared with that for singleton pregnancies. This risk is significantly higher in monochorionic (11.6%) than dichorionic (5%) pregnancies. Though most of this excess risk for monochorionic twins compared to dichorionic twins occurs before 24 weeks, with the suggestion that survival rates are similar after this gestation, there is still increased risk of intrauterine demise with structurally normal well-grown monochorionic twins with no TTTS after 32 weeks compared to dichorionic twins.[4]

Specific to monochorionic twin pregnancy is the complication of twin-to-twin transfusion syndrome (TTTS), twin reversed arterial perfusion (TRAP) sequence and cord entanglement for monoamniotic twins.

TWIN-TO-TWIN TRANSFUSION SYNDROME

TTTS is caused by an imbalance in the haemodynamic communication between the circulation of the twins at the placenta, resulting in an anaemic donor twin with oligohydramnios (stuck twin) and a polycythaemic recipient with polyhydramnios and cardiac overload. TTTS complicates 15% of monochorionic pregnancies and if left untreated leads to perinatal mortality in 90% of cases. There is a 50% risk of neurological impairment due to prematurity or the intrauterine demise of one twin.[5]

There are three types of communication between the two circulations at the placenta. Artery-to-artery (AAA) and vein-to-vein anastomoses (VVA) are superficial on the chorionic plate and mediate bidirectional flow across the placenta, with AAA thought to be protective against TTTS. Artery-to-vein anastomoses (AVA) are deep in the placenta and mediate unidirectional flow across the placenta, and an imbalance in this flow is thought to be pathophysiologic for TTTS.

TTTS usually manifests in the second trimester (rarely in the early third trimester) and can be staged using the Quintero staging system (Table 3.3). Prognosis is better in early TTTS (stages I and II) compared with advanced disease (stages III and IV). Though this staging is useful for consistent description of the complication and outcomes, it does not always denote a logical order of progression of disease. There is an 80% risk of perinatal mortality and 15–20% risk of brain injury in survivors.[6]

Fetoscopic laser ablation of the intertwin anastomoses on the chorionic plate should be the preferred treatment of severe TTTS (stages II, III and IV) before 26 weeks, as demonstrated by the Eurofetus trial, rather than amnioreduction or septostomy, because laser ablation corrects the pathophysiologic cause of the disease. Laser ablation is usually for stages II and III, with the attendant risks of preterm pre-labour rupture of membranes, preterm delivery, vaginal bleeding, abruption, chorioamnionitis, limb ischaemia, bowel atresia, recurrence of TTTS and loss of one or both twins. With laser ablation there is a 30–50% risk of perinatal mortality and a 5–20% risk of long-term neurologic handicap, with a 50% chance of intact survival of both twins.[5,6]

Surveillance should continue after laser ablation because there is a 14% risk of persisting or recurring TTTS and reversed TTTS. The optimal timing for the

Table 3.3 Quintero staging system for twin-to-twin transfusion syndrome

Stage	Classification
I	There is a discrepancy in amniotic fluid volume, with oligohydramnios of a maximum vertical pocket (MVP) $\leq$ 2 cm in one sac and polyhydramnios in the other sac (MVP $\geq$ 8 cm). The bladder of the donor twin is visible and Doppler studies are normal.
II	The bladder of the donor twin is not visible (during length of examination, usually around 1 hour) but Doppler studies are not critically abnormal.
III	Doppler studies are critically abnormal in either twin and are characterized as abnormal or reversed end-diastolic velocities in the umbilical artery, reverse flow in the ductus venosus or pulsatile umbilical venous flow.
IV	Ascites, pericardial or pleural effusion, scalp oedema or overt hydrops present.
V	One or both babies are dead.

delivery of treated TTTS pregnancies is uncertain, but most of the pregnancies in published trials and case reviews were delivered at 33–34 weeks.

Management options for severe TTTS after 26 weeks include delivery, with the attendant risks of prematurity and perinatal morbidity and mortality; amnioreduction, with attendant risks of preterm labour; and laser ablation. However, laser ablation becomes technically more difficult to perform with advancing gestation. Stage I TTTS may best be managed expectantly, because 75% of cases remain stable or regress and survival rates exceed 80%.

DISCORDANT GROWTH

Discordant growth presents management dilemmas particularly for monochorionic twins. Discordant growth is defined as a 15–25% difference in estimated fetal weight between the fetuses. It is associated with chromosomal anomalies, placental dysfunction, genetic disorders, velamentous cord insertion and single umbilical artery in both dichorionic and monochorionic pregnancies. A major cause for growth discordance in monochorionic pregnancy is TTTS. Discordant crown–rump length (CRL) of $\geq$ 10mm is predictive of twin pregnancies at increased risk of discordant growth and weight, though not of TTTS.

Monitoring is by serial ultrasound estimation of fetal weight and growth velocity. Doppler assessment of the umbilical and middle cerebral arteries and of the ductus venosus is carried out as for singleton pregnancies, with the aim of prolonging the pregnancy where possible in order to reduce the risk of prematurity and associated neonatal complications.

The management principle of selective growth restriction is to balance the risk of fetal death of the growth-restricted twin (with expectant care) against the risk of iatrogenic prematurity to the well-grown twin (with early delivery to salvage the smaller twin). In addition, there is the significant risk of neurological injury and death of the co-twin if one twin in a monochorionic pregnancy dies.

For both dichorionic and monochorionic twins, delivery by caesarean section after the administration of steroids should be considered after 28 weeks if a viable weight has been attained by the smaller twin, the umbilical artery Doppler shows reversed end-diastolic flow, and the ductus venosus shows abnormal waveforms (usually a reversed A wave). In situations of imminent demise of the severely growth-restricted non-viable monochorionic twin and the attendant risk to the co-twin, cord occlusion of the former or laser ablation of chorionic plate anastomoses to ensure intact survival of the healthy co-twin is a valid option.

MONOFETAL DEATH

Monofetal death occurs in 3–6% of twin pregnancies. The attendant risk from this event is dependent on the gestation and chorionicity. The risk is higher in the second and third trimesters and in monochorionic pregnancies. These risks

Table 3.4	Twin pregnancy risks following monofetal death	
Risk	*Monochorionic*	*Dichorionic*
Co-twin demise	12%	4%
Neurological injury	18%	1%
Preterm delivery (< 34 weeks)	68%	57%

include co-twin demise, neurological injury, end-organ failure and preterm delivery, which can be iatrogenic or spontaneous (Table 3.4). Structural abnormalities associated with neurological injury and end-organ failure include multicystic encephalomalacia, microcephaly, hydranencephaly, porencephaly, hydrocephalus, haemorrhagic lesions of the white matter, gastrointestinal bowel atresia and bilateral renal cortical necrosis. The 'vanishing twin' phenomenon, with loss of one twin in the first trimester, is relatively common and has a good prognosis for the surviving dichorionic co-twin.

In dichorionic twins, the prognosis for the surviving twin is good, with prematurity the main risk. In the absence of other complications, conservative management with fortnightly growth scans and Doppler studies, steroids for lung maturity and delivery at 37 weeks is recommended.

The risks of co-twin neurological injury and demise in monochorionic twins could be as a result of haemodynamic shifts across placental anastomoses leading to hypovolaemia and hypoperfusion and the transplacental passage of thrombotic material from the dead to the living twin with resulting ischaemia and infarction. These would have occurred before the monofetal demise is detected, and thus there would seem to be no benefit in immediate delivery of the surviving twin, which could worsen risks due to prematurity.[7]

Conservative management is by weekly ultrasound and Doppler studies of the middle cerebral artery to detect fetal anaemia and other signs of monofetal death sequelae that might take 3–4 weeks to manifest. Fetal MRI to assess for cerebral lesions is performed 2–3 weeks after monofetal demise and might be repeated later if the demise occurred in the early third trimester. Late termination would then be an option if brain lesions are detected. In the absence of evidence of neurological lesions, delivery is best at term, either vaginally or by caesarean section.

SELECTIVE FETAL REDUCTION

Selective fetal reduction is the procedure by which one or more fetuses, identified with genetic, chromosomal or structural abnormalities, is terminated. For dichorionic pregnancies this is usually by intracardiac potassium chloride or lidocaine. This is usually in the first or early second trimester following counselling for severe fetal abnormalities detected by that gestation. In order to avoid reducing the wrong fetus in situations with abnormal karyotype but no evident structural abnormality to identify the fetus, accurate fetal mapping at screening must be followed by accurate mapping at diagnostic testing and feticide by a fetal medicine specialist.[2]

For abnormalities identified after the early second trimester, consideration must be given to the timing of the feticide. Although there is increased risk of miscarriage and preterm delivery after feticide at later gestations, earlier feticide could be attended by total pregnancy loss. On the other hand, waiting till after viability to improve the chance of survival of the non-affected fetus increases the risk of the live birth of an anomalous fetus should spontaneous preterm delivery supervene.[4]

For monochorionic pregnancies, the indications for selective fetal reduction include heterokaryotypic chromosomal abnormalities, discordant structural anomalies, severe discordant growth restriction and TRAP sequence. Selective reduction is by cord occlusion (bipolar cord occlusion, umbilical cord ligation or laser coagulation) or by intrafetal ablation of intra-abdominal umbilical or aorto-pelvic vessels (using radiofrequency ablation, interstitial laser ablation or mono-polar thermocoagulation).

HIGHER-ORDER MULTIPLE PREGNANCIES

Higher-order multiple pregnancies have much higher risks of complications. The perinatal outcome is significantly affected by high rates of preterm delivery and low birth weight, leading to higher mortality and cerebral palsy rates. In addition, there are higher rates of maternal complications such as gestational diabetes, hypertension in pregnancy and bleeding.

As the majority of higher-order multiple pregnancies (≥ 3) result from assisted reproduction technology, the risk of multiple pregnancy should be reduced by conservative use of ovarian stimulation, and consideration given to transferring only a single embryo. Also, couples with higher-order multiple pregnancies should be counselled and offered multifetal pregnancy reduction to twins (MFPR). MFPR is optimally done at 11–14 weeks, after screening for chromosomal and gross structural abnormalities and the risk period for first-trimester pregnancy loss has passed. The ethical dilemmas associated with MFPR of lower-order multiple pregnancies (twins and triplets) are beyond the scope of this chapter.[8]

Antenatal care

Given the increased risk to both mothers and babies, women with multiple pregnancies need more contact with healthcare professionals than women with singleton pregnancies. Their care should be provided by a specialist with experi-ence in managing multiple pregnancy. Increasingly this care is being provided in specialist multidisciplinary multiple-pregnancy clinics. There should be care path-ways that allow for referral to the regional fetal medicine unit.

Indications for referral to a tertiary-level fetal medicine unit include mono-chorionic monoamniotic twin pregnancies, monochorionic monoamniotic triplet pregnancies, monochorionic diamniotic triplet pregnancies, dichorionic diamniotic triplet pregnancies and any pregnancy complicated by discordant fetal growth, fetal anomaly, discordant fetal death or TTTS.[2]

A first-trimester ultrasound scan is used to confirm multiple gestation, date the pregnancy and determine chorionicity and amnionicity. The presence of two separate placental masses confirms dichorionic twin pregnancy. If there is one placental mass, the presence of the lambda sign confirms dichorionicity while the T sign is seen in monochorionic pairs. Other sonographic markers of chorionicity are intertwin membrane thickness ($<$ 2 mm indicative of monochorionic twins) and discordant sex of the fetuses. Where chorionicity is in doubt, such as can happen if the first scan is in the second trimester, the patient should be referred to a fetal medicine specialist. If chorionicity cannot be determined, the pregnancy should be managed as a monochorionic pregnancy.

The pregnancy is usually dated according to the CRL of the larger twin if the equivalent gestational age is between 11 and 14 weeks. Some studies suggest that using the CRL of the smaller twin or the mean CRL to date the pregnancy does not significantly differ from using the CRL of the larger twin. Significant discrepancy of intertwin CRL of more than 9.8 mm at 11–14 weeks increases the risk of major growth delay, likely secondary to aneuploidy.

Screening for Down's syndrome for twin pregnancies is best performed by combining ultrasound assessment of the nuchal translucency (NT) and serum screening by determination of free β-hCG and PAPP-A levels. For dichorionic twins, each twin is given an initial risk based on the NT which is then multiplied by the likelihood ratio derived from the serum markers. For monochorionic twins the risk generated by an average NT is multiplied by the likelihood ratio derived from the serum markers, giving a single risk estimate for both twins. This screening method would give a 72% detection rate for a 5% false-positive rate. For triplet pregnancies, individual NT and maternal age can be used to screen for risk of Down's syndrome, with higher false-positive rates. It is important to specifically map the fetuses during dating and screening in order to assign the correct risk to each fetus. A risk of 1 : 150 or higher is considered high, as for singleton pregnancies.[2]

If there is high risk of Down's syndrome from screening, increased risk of chromosomal abnormalities due to the presence of structural abnormalities or a desire for prenatal testing due to family history of monogenic disorders, the pregnancy should be referred to a tertiary fetal medicine centre for further counselling and invasive diagnostic testing. Prenatal testing in multiple pregnancies presents challenges regarding making the decision to proceed with a test, technical difficulties with invasive testing and the subsequent management of the test result, including selective feticide. The risk of fetal loss is higher compared to singleton pregnancies, with a similar risk of 3.2% before 20–24 weeks for both chorionic villus sampling and amniocentesis.

Chorionic villus sampling of the separate placentas in dichorionic pregnancies or the shared placenta in monochorionic pregnancies can be done between

11 weeks 0 days and 14 weeks 6 days. In dichorionic pregnancies with fused placentas there is the risk of contamination of samples with tissue from the other placenta, and of inadequate sampling in a bid to avoid contamination and sampling of the wrong placental mass.

Amniocentesis is the gold standard for both mono- and dichorionic twin pregnancies. Both twin sacs are sampled by either a single- or a double-puncture technique. For a single approach the proximal sac is accessed first, followed by advancement of the needle into the second sac. There is a small risk of contamination associated with this approach. With monochorionic twins, it is acceptable to sample only one sac. However, rarely, the twins could be heterokaryotypic, and it is therefore recommended to sample both sacs by the double technique especially if there is discordant structural abnormality or growth restriction. Amniocentesis should be the preferred prenatal test for triplet pregnancies.

A scan of fetal anatomy is routine at 18–20 weeks. Monochorionic twins should be scanned every 2 weeks from 16 weeks till 24 weeks to detect TTTS and then every 2–3 weeks until delivery in order to detect fetal growth restriction. Triplets should have a similar monitoring schedule. Dichorionic twins should have growth scans every 3–4 weeks from 20 weeks till delivery.

It is usual to perform a full blood count at 20 weeks, because of the increased incidence of anaemia, and to offer early iron and folic acid supplementation. The full blood count is repeated at 28 weeks as a matter of routine. 75 mg aspirin should be offered from 12 weeks to delivery if there are other risk factors for hypertension such as first pregnancy, family history of pre-eclampsia, BMI > 35 kg/m^2 or age 40 years or older.

Although there is increased risk of preterm delivery with twin pregnancies, cervical length monitoring, fibronectin testing and home uterine activity monitoring should not be used routinely to predict the risk of preterm delivery. Similarly, home bed rest, intramuscular or vaginal progesterone, cervical cerclage and oral tocolytics should not be routinely used to prevent preterm birth. Single or multiple untargeted (routine) administration of steroids for lung maturation should not be offered. None of these measures has been shown to be of fetal or maternal benefit.[2]

Mode and timing of delivery

The mode of delivery of twin pregnancies will depend on chorionicity, amnionicity, gestation, the experience of the attending clinician, the presentation of the first twin and the presence of any other maternal and fetal complications such as previous caesarean section, severe pre-eclampsia, fetal growth restriction, TTTS, etc. For uncomplicated dichorionic and monochorionic diamniotic twins with cephalic presentation of the first twin, vaginal delivery is recommended.

Some would recommend caesarean section for the delivery of monochorionic diamniotic twins because of the risk of acute transfusion in labour, although the evidence base for this is unclear. Breech presentation of the first twin would be an indication for delivery by caesarean section because of the risks of breech delivery to that twin and of interlocking twins.

Monoamniotic twins should be delivered by caesarean section. For triplets and higher-order multiple pregnancies, caesarean section is recommended.

If there are no indications for earlier delivery, dichorionic twins should be delivered at 38 weeks gestation and monochorionic diamniotic twins at 36–37 weeks. It is recommended to deliver monoamniotic twins at 32–34 weeks because of the risk of cord entanglement leading to fetal demise. Triplet pregnancies should be delivered after 35 weeks.[9]

The timing, mode and management of delivery should be discussed antenatally. This discussion should ideally take place at 34–36 weeks for dichorionic twins and at 32–34 weeks for monochorionic twins.[2]

Intrapartum care

Twins should be delivered in a consultant-led delivery unit with an experienced obstetrician skilled in the delivery of twins, experienced midwives, and an anaesthetist in attendance. Depending on the gestation, type of twin and any antenatal complications there should be availability of neonatal cots with paediatricians/ neonatologists attending the delivery. The position and presentation of the twins should be confirmed by ultrasound on admission.

The management of labour should be discussed again on admission, with questions by the couple answered and their preferences noted. This discussion should cover the personnel who will be present both during labour and at delivery, the need for continuous electronic fetal monitoring and pain relief options, including the possible benefit of epidural to help with manoeuvres that might be needed particularly with the delivery of the second twin. These possible manoeuvres should also be briefly explained.

Elective delivery can be induced with prostaglandins, amniotomy and oxytocin infusion. In labour, an intravenous line should be sited, with blood samples obtained to assess haemoglobin level and for crossmatching later if needed. Continuous electronic fetal heart monitoring with the use of a specific twin monitor that can record both fetal heart rates simultaneously on the same trace is necessary. It is important to ensure that the monitor is not recording the same fetal heart rate twice, and this can be facilitated by applying a fetal scalp electrode to the leading twin once membranes are ruptured. The monitoring of the second twin should continue after delivery of the first twin.

After the delivery of the first twin, the lie and presentation of the second twin should be ascertained by abdominal and vaginal examination. The use of an ultrasound machine can help with this. If the lie is longitudinal with a cephalic or breech presentation, the delivery should proceed. Amniotomy of the second sac should be performed with care taken to avoid cord prolapse. Delivery should then proceed as routine. Oxytocin augmentation might be needed at this stage to ensure adequate contractions.

Traditionally, a delivery interval of 30 minutes between twins has been advocated, but if the fetal heart monitoring is satisfactory and delivery is progressing satisfactorily, strict adherence to this interval might not be required. The cord of each twin should be identified and double-clamped, and cord blood obtained for blood gases.

If the lie is not longitudinal, version abdominally to correct this either to cephalic presentation (preferable) or breech is performed. Occasionally, internal podalic version, where the feet are grasped and the breech brought down to the vagina, can be attempted. It might be beneficial to attempt this in the theatre with immediate recourse to emergency caesarean section if it fails or there is fetal distress.

Active management of the third stage is needed because of the increased risk of postpartum haemorrhage. This is achieved with the administration of oxytocin and/or ergometrine with the delivery of the shoulders of the second twin and an oxytocin infusion.

Key summary points

- A first-trimester ultrasound scan should confirm multiple pregnancy, date the pregnancy and determine chorionicity and amnionicity.
- Invasive diagnostic testing should be carried out by fetal medicine specialists.
- There should be care pathways that allow for referral to the regional fetal medicine unit.
- Monochorionic twins should be scanned fortnightly from 16 to 24 weeks and then every 2–3 weeks, and dichorionic twins every 3–4 weeks from 20 weeks.
- Fetoscopic laser ablation of the intertwin anastomoses on the chorionic plate should be the preferred treatment for severe TTTS.

References

1. Office for National Statistics. *Births in England and Wales by Characteristics of Birth 2, 2011.* London: ONS, 2013.

2. National Institute for Health and Care Excellence (NICE). *Multiple Pregnancy: the Management of Twin and Triplet Pregnancies in the Antenatal Period.* NICE Clinical Guideline CG129. London: NICE, 2011.

3. Glinianaia SV, Rankin J, Wright C. Congenital anomalies in twins: a register-based study. *Hum Reprod* 2008; 23: 1306–11.

4. Engineer N, Fisk N. Multiple pregnancy. In Rodeck CH, Whittle MJ, eds. *Fetal Medicine: Basic Science and Clinical Practice.* Edinburgh: Churchill Livingstone, 2009, pp. 649–77.

5. Royal College of Obstetricians and Gynaecologists. *Management of Monochorionic Twin Pregnancy.* Green-top Guideline No. 51. London: RCOG, 2008.

6. Chalouhi GE, Essaoui M, Stirnemann J, *et al.* Laser therapy for twin-to-twin transfusion syndrome (TTTS). *Prenat Diagn* 2011; 31: 637–46.

7. Ong SS, Zamora J, Khan KS, Kilby MD. Prognosis for the co-twin following single-twin death: a systematic review. *BJOG* 2006; 113: 992–8.

8. Consensus views arising from the 50th Study Group: multiple pregnancy. In Kilby M, Baker P, Critchley H, Field D, eds. *Multiple Pregnancy.* London: RCOG Press, 2006, pp. 283–6

9. Lee YM. Delivery of twins. *Semin Perinatol* 2012; 36: 195–200.

4 Hypertensive disorders in pregnancy

Fiona Fairlie

Introduction

Hypertensive disorders are the most common medical complications encountered by obstetricians, affecting 10–15% of pregnancies. Worldwide, they contribute significantly to maternal and perinatal mortality and morbidity. The presenting signs and symptoms of hypertensive disorders are varied and often subtle in onset. In the UK, eclampsia, HELLP syndrome and the neurological, pulmonary, hepatic, renal and haematological complications of severe pre-eclampsia are relatively uncommon. Most obstetricians and anaesthetists have little first-hand experience of these complications. Consequently it is not surprising that they may be unrecognized until an advanced stage, and/or inappropriate treatment may be administered.

This chapter incorporates recommendations made by the National Institute for Health and Care Excellence (NICE) in its 2010 guideline for the management of hypertensive disorders in pregnancy.[1]

Definitions (NICE 2010)[1]

Chronic hypertension – Hypertension present at booking visit or before 20 weeks, or that is being treated at time of referral to maternity services. It may be primary or secondary in aetiology.

Eclampsia – Convulsive condition associated with pre-eclampsia.

Gestational hypertension – New hypertension presenting after 20 weeks without significant proteinuria.

Pre-eclampsia – New hypertension presenting after 20 weeks with significant proteinuria.

Pre-eclampsia may be mild or severe. Severe pre-eclampsia is pre-eclampsia with severe hypertension and/or with symptoms, and/or biochemical and/or haematological impairment. Clinical symptoms include:

Antenatal Disorders for the MRCOG and Beyond, Second Edition, ed. Dilly Anumba and Shehnaaz Jivraj. Published by Cambridge University Press. © Cambridge University Press 2016.

- severe headache
- loss of vision, double vision, papilloedema
- epigastric pain
- vomiting
- clonus
- liver tenderness

Pre-eclampsia may present with proteinuria without a significant rise in blood pressure (10% of cases).

DEGREES OF HYPERTENSION

Mild – Diastolic blood pressure 90–99 mmHg, systolic blood pressure 140–149 mmHg.

Moderate – Diastolic blood pressure 100–109 mmHg, systolic blood pressure 150–159 mmHg.

Severe – Diastolic blood pressure $\geq$ 110 mmHg, systolic blood pressure $\geq$ 160 mmHg.

SIGNIFICANT PROTEINURIA

Urinary protein : creatinine ratio > 30 mg/mmol or a validated 24-hour urine collection result > 300 mg protein.

MEASUREMENT OF BLOOD PRESSURE

During normal pregnancy, blood pressure falls in the first trimester following a decrease in systemic vascular resistance. On average, the diastolic blood pressure is 15 mmHg lower in the second trimester compared with before pregnancy. Blood pressure increases in the third trimester to reach pre-pregnancy levels by term.

The measurement of blood pressure is fundamental in the diagnosis and management of the hypertensive disorders of pregnancy. Before measuring blood pressure manually, the woman should be rested and sitting at a 45-degree angle. The blood pressure cuff should be of the appropriate size, with the air bladder covering at least three-quarters of the circumference of the upper arm. Korotkoff phase 5 is the appropriate measurement of diastolic blood pressure, as this corresponds more closely to intra-arterial pressure, is more reproducible and is more closely related to outcome.

Automated methods of measuring blood pressure are in common use. They may underestimate blood pressure readings in pre-eclampsia, especially at higher levels, and their accuracy should be confirmed by comparison with manual sphygmomanometry.

MEASUREMENT OF PROTEINURIA (NICE 2010)[1]

- In normal pregnancy, up to 300 mg of total protein may be excreted in the urine of healthy women in 24 hours.
- An automated reagent-strip reading device or spot urinary protein : creatinine ratio (PCR) should be used to estimate proteinuria in secondary care.
- If an automated reagent-strip reading device shows ≥ 1+ proteinuria, a spot urinary PCR or 24-hour urine collection should be used to quantify proteinuria.

Why is hypertensive disease in pregnancy important?

MATERNAL MORTALITY AND MORBIDITY

Hypertensive disease is a major cause of maternal death worldwide. Most adverse outcomes are due to pre-eclampsia/eclampsia/HELLP syndrome. Although the UK mortality from hypertensive disease has fallen significantly since the first Confidential Enquiry into Maternal Deaths in 1952–54, there has been little decline over the last 30 years. Of 19 deaths in the 2006–08 enquiry, almost all were associated with substandard care, and in more than half this was classified as major.[2] Intracranial haemorrhage secondary to severe hypertension was the most common cause of death, highlighting the importance of administering effective antihypertensive therapy.

Hypertensive disease may be associated with severe maternal morbidity. A UK study of eclampsia conducted between February 2005 and February 2006 identified 214 cases.[3] No women in the study died. However, there was considerable morbidity: 26% had recurrent fits; 56% were admitted to intensive care or obstetric high-dependency units for between 1 and 9 days; 10% were reported to have other severe morbidity after the eclamptic episode.

PERINATAL MORTALITY AND MORBIDITY

Hypertensive disorders carry a significant risk to the fetus and neonate. In a recent UK survey of perinatal deaths (2011) hypertensive disorders of pregnancy contributed 5.9% of all stillbirths.[4] The perinatal mortality rate in the UK eclampsia study was 59/1000 births (95% CI 32–98).[3]

Mortality and morbidity are mainly due to preterm delivery and/or fetal growth restriction. Between 8% and 10% of all preterm births are due to hypertensive disorders. In women with pre-eclampsia, 20–25% of preterm births and 14–19% of term births are below the 10th centile of birth weight for gestation.

Pre-conception care

Ideally women considered to be at risk of hypertensive disorders in pregnancy should be seen before conception. This provides an opportunity to optimize the management of pre-existing medical conditions and convert medications to those least likely to cause fetal harm. Women can be given information about the risks of developing pre-eclampsia and/or fetal growth restriction and offered prophylaxis.

Women who are likely to benefit from pre-conception care include those with:

- previous pre-eclampsia
- chronic hypertension
- chronic kidney disease
- cardiac disease
- antiphospholipid syndrome
- systemic lupus erythematosus

Antihypertensive medication

The purpose of antihypertensive therapy is to protect the woman from the effects of hypertension, especially cerebral haemorrhage and eclampsia. Elevated blood pressure should be treated regardless of its aetiology. By effectively lowering blood pressure, antihypertensive medication allows the pregnancy to advance and reduces the risk of medical interventions, including hospital admission, caesarean section and premature delivery. However, antihypertensive medication does not alter the progress of the disease in pre-eclampsia, nor does it reduce the risk of developing superimposed pre-eclampsia in essential hypertension.

Above a mean arterial blood pressure of 125–130 mmHg, there is a loss of maternal cerebral autoregulation. To protect the mother, hypertension should be treated to keep the systolic pressure less than 150 mmHg and the diastolic less than 100 mmHg. Lowering blood pressure may cause under-perfusion of the placenta. Whether there is benefit to the fetus in 'less tight' control of diastolic blood pressure (aiming for a level of 100 mmHg), compared with 'tight' control (aiming for 85 mmHg), has recently been investigated in the CHIPS trial. There was no significant difference with respect to the risk of pregnancy loss, high-level neonatal care or overall maternal complications, although less tight control was associated with a significantly higher frequency of severe maternal hypertension.[5]

The most common antihypertensive drugs used to treat hypertension during pregnancy are shown in Table 4.1. Oral labetalol is the initial treatment of choice for new-onset hypertension in pregnancy unless contraindicated (e.g. asthma). Intravenous agents can be employed if blood pressure is not controlled with oral agents, or if the woman is unable to tolerate oral agents for any reason.

Labetalol is the only antihypertensive agent licensed for treatment in pregnancy, although the other drugs listed have been used extensively in pregnancy and appear to be safe for mother and fetus. Beta-blockers such as atenolol are relatively contraindicated in pregnancy due to their association with fetal growth restriction. Methyldopa should be avoided postpartum because of its association with depression.

Table 4.1 Antihypertensive agents commonly used in pregnancy

Drug	Action	Dosage	Side effects	Contraindications
Labetalol	α and β blocker	Oral: 200 mg tds to 400 mg qds Intravenous: bolus dose 50 mg given slowly followed by continuous infusion up to 160 mg/h	Bradycardia Bronchospasm Scalp tingling	Asthma Phaeochromocytoma
Nifedipine	Calcium channel antagonist	Oral:10 mg bd to 20 mg qds	Headache Flushing Tachycardia Oedema Lethargy	Aortic stenosis Liver disease Avoid before 20 weeks gestation (NICE 2010)[1]
Methyldopa	Central action	Oral: 250 mg tds to 1 g tds	Tiredness Postural hypotension Depression Headaches Dry mouth Gastrointestinal disturbances	Phaeochromocytoma Liver disease Depression Avoid postpartum
Hydralazine	Vasodilator	Oral: 25mg tds to 75mg qds Intravenous: bolus 5–10 mg in sodium chloride administered slowly over 10–20 minutes followed by a continuous infusion of 5–20 mg/h	Tachycardia Palpitations Flushing Fluid retention	

ANTIHYPERTENSIVE MEDICATION AND BREASTFEEDING

Labetalol, nifedipine, enalapril, captopril, atenolol and metoprolol have no known adverse effects on breastfed babies. Postnatally, women with chronic hypertension usually revert to their pre-pregnancy medication.

Outpatient management of hypertensive disorders in pregnancy

Outpatient management of women with mild or moderate hypertension was introduced in the early 1980s.[6] Obstetric day-care units provide a comprehensive assessment of maternal and fetal wellbeing with senior clinician review. They offer safe, effective and economically sound management when appropriately targeted.[7,8] Furthermore women prefer outpatient care to hospital admission. The frequency of day-care appointments will depend on the woman's medical/obstetric history, results of recent maternal/fetal monitoring and gestation.

APEC (Action on Pre-eclampsia charity, action-on-pre-eclampsia.org.uk), the Royal College of Obstetricians and Gynaecologists (RCOG) and NICE have collaborated to provide the PRECOG guidelines for community midwives to detect early signs of pre-eclampsia and refer to day-care or hospital admission.[9]

These guidelines advise **hospital referral** if:

- Diastolic blood pressure $\geq$ 90 mmHg or systolic blood pressure is $\geq$ 160 mmHg.
- 2+ or more proteinuria on dipstick or $\geq$ 1+ on dipstick with significant symptoms.
- Epigastric pain even if BP is $<$ 90 mmHg and trace or no proteinuria.

The urgency of hospital referral depends on the blood pressure level, degree of proteinuria and presence/absence of symptoms.

Immediate hospital admission is advised if:

- Diastolic blood pressure is $\geq$ 110 mmHg and new proteinuria $\geq$ 1+ on dipstick.
- Diastolic blood pressure is $\geq$ 90 mmHg and new proteinuria $\geq$ 1+ on dipstick with significant symptoms (including epigastric pain, vomiting, headache, visual disturbances, reduced fetal movements, small-for-gestational-age fetus).
- Systolic blood pressure is $\geq$ 170 mmHg.

In 2009 PRECOG2 was published.[9] This guideline is for midwives working in day-care units and advises on how to care for women diagnosed with pre-eclampsia.

Management of chronic hypertension

Women with chronic hypertension should be advised to have their blood pressure control and medication reviewed before they conceive. Once pregnant, the need for antihypertensive medication should be reassessed. These women often exhibit the same fall in blood pressure as seen in normal pregnancy, and they may not require therapy until the second or third trimester.

Hypertension presenting for the first time in early pregnancy should not be assumed to be essential until secondary causes such as renal, adrenal and cardiac have been excluded.

There is no drug of preference for the management of chronic hypertension in pregnancy. However, angiotensin-converting enzyme (ACE) inhibitors, angiotensin II receptor blockers and chlorothiazide are associated with a risk of congenital anomalies and should be avoided. Women planning to conceive and taking any of these agents should be advised to change to medications such as methyldopa or labetalol prior to conception.

For women with uncomplicated chronic hypertension, the aim is to keep blood pressure less than 150 mmHg systolic and between 80 and 100 mmHg diastolic.

If there is target-organ damage due to hypertension (e.g. kidney disease), systolic blood pressure should be kept below 140 mmHg and diastolic between 80 and 90 mmHg.

Women with secondary chronic hypertension should be managed in conjunction with their physician.

Chronic hypertension is associated with a risk of superimposed pre-eclampsia, fetal growth restriction and placental abruption. An individual plan should be made for the frequency of antenatal assessments depending on medical and obstetric history and any additional risk factors for adverse outcome. Measurement of blood pressure and urinalysis should be every 2–4 weeks from 20 weeks onwards. At 28–30 weeks and 32–34 weeks ultrasound measurements of fetal growth and amniotic fluid volume and umbilical artery Doppler should be undertaken. If the results are normal, further ultrasound assessment is not indicated unless the clinical situation deteriorates. Fetal cardiotocography should be carried out if there are concerns about fetal activity. If blood pressure can be maintained below 160/110 mmHg and there is no evidence of fetal compromise or superimposed pre-eclampsia, then pregnancy can be prolonged to at least 37 weeks.

During labour, antenatal antihypertensive treatment should be continued, with the aim of keeping systolic pressure less than 150 mmHg. If blood pressure is stable and less than 150/100 mmHg then it is not necessary to limit the duration of second stage. Continuous fetal heart rate monitoring is recommended. After birth, ergometrine, including Syntometrine (Alliance), should be avoided, as these drugs can further increase the blood pressure.

After birth, maternal blood pressure should be measured daily for the first 2 days and at least once between the third and fifth postnatal day, with the aim of keeping the level below 140/90 mmHg. If antihypertensive medication is required, methyldopa should be avoided because of its association with depression. Alternative agents include labetalol, nifedipine, atenolol and enalapril. Blood pressure control should be reviewed 6–8 weeks postpartum by the woman's general practitioner.

Management of gestational hypertension

ANTEPARTUM CARE

Women with mild or moderate hypertension (blood pressure < 160/110 mmHg) can be safely managed as outpatients. At each antenatal visit, urine should be tested for proteinuria with either an automated reagent-strip reading device or urinary PCR. Moderate hypertension (150/100 mmHg to 159/109 mmHg) should be treated to maintain systolic pressure below 150 mmHg and diastolic pressure 80–100 mmHg. Once treatment has been initiated, blood pressure should be measured at least twice a week.

Women with moderate hypertension should have blood tests for renal function, electrolytes, full blood count, transaminases and bilirubin at initial diagnosis. Repeat testing is not required unless proteinuria develops.

In the event of severe hypertension, the woman should be admitted to hospital and started on antihypertensive medication (or medication increased) to maintain systolic pressure below 150 mmHg and diastolic pressure 80–100 mmHg. Blood pressure should be measured at least four times a day and urine tested for protein daily with either an automated reagent-strip reading device or urinary PCR. Blood tests for renal function, electrolytes, full blood count, transaminases and bilirubin should be taken at admission and weekly thereafter. Once severe gestational hypertension has been controlled, outpatient management can be instituted with twice-weekly blood pressure and urine testing and weekly blood tests.

Women who present before 32 weeks with mild hypertension or who are high risk for pre-eclampsia should be advised to have their blood pressure measured and urine tested twice weekly.

There are no studies of fetal surveillance in populations that include only women with gestational hypertension. An individual plan for fetal monitoring should be made depending on gestation at diagnosis, severity of hypertension and any previous history of pre-eclampsia, stillbirth or a small-for-dates baby. Ultrasound examinations for fetal growth, amniotic fluid assessment and umbilical artery Doppler velocimetry should not normally be repeated more frequently than every two weeks unless the clinical situation changes or the results are abnormal. For women with mild or moderate gestational hypertension fetal cardiotocography is only indicated if fetal activity is abnormal. If hypertension is severe and conservative management is planned, then fetal cardiotocography should be at least once a week, and more often if the clinical situation changes.

TIMING OF DELIVERY

Pregnancy can be prolonged to reach fetal maturity at 37 weeks if blood pressure is less than 160/110 mmHg with or without treatment and there are no concerns about fetal wellbeing. After 37 weeks, the woman can be offered induction of labour. The HYPITAT trial demonstrated that induction of labour in women with gestational hypertension or pre-eclampsia at term resulted in less progression to severe disease, without a higher caesarean section rate.[10]

CARE IN LABOUR

Blood pressure should be measured hourly if hypertension is mild or moderate, and continually if severe. Antihypertensive medication should be continued. It is not necessary to limit the duration of second stage unless hypertension is severe and unresponsive to treatment. Oxytocin should be administered for active management of third stage. Ergometrine/Syntometrine are contraindicated, as these agents can produce an acute rise in blood pressure.

POSTNATAL CARE

Blood pressure should be recorded daily for the first 2 days and at least once between 3 and 5 days after birth. Before discharge to community care, blood pressure should be stable below 150/100 mmHg. On transfer to community care, a plan of management should be documented including frequency of blood pressure monitoring and when to reduce/stop antihypertensive treatment. Antihypertensive medication can be reduced once blood pressure falls below 130/80 mmHg. Women who did not require treatment for hypertension before birth will require medication postpartum if their blood pressure rises above 149/99 mmHg.

A general practitioner review should be advised for women who require antihypertensive medication at two weeks post birth. Women with gestational hypertension should be offered a medical review 6–8 weeks postpartum. This is an opportunity to review blood pressure control, and to discuss contraception and the implications of gestational hypertension for future pregnancies and long-term health (Table 4.2). Women with persistent hypertension requiring medication eight weeks postpartum should be referred to a specialist for investigation.

Long-term significance of hypertension in pregnancy

Pregnancy may be considered as a vascular stress test. Women who develop gestational hypertension or pre-eclampsia are at increased risk of developing hypertension and its complications in later life. Women should be informed of the risk of recurrent hypertensive disease in pregnancy and lifetime risk of cardiovascular and kidney disease (Table 4.2).

There is an association between pre-eclampsia and maternal thrombophilia. However, there is insufficient evidence of benefit to recommend routine screening for thrombophilia in women who have had pre-eclampsia.

Pre-eclampsia

AETIOLOGY AND PATHOGENESIS

Although advances have been made in understanding the pathophysiology of pre-eclampsia, the initiating event(s) is unknown.[11] The pathophysiological features of pre-eclampsia include systemic inflammation, oxidative stress, altered levels of angiogenic factors, increased vascular reactivity, endothelial dysfunction and activation, insulin resistance and dyslipidaemia. Many of these changes are seen in normal pregnancy but to a lesser degree.

Table 4.2 Long-term health risks (NICE 2010)[1]

Future risk	Hypertensive disorder		
	Gestational hypertension	Pre-eclampsia	Severe pre-eclampsia, HELLP syndrome or eclampsia
Gestational hypertension in future pregnancy	Risk ranges from about 1 in 6 (16%) to about 1 in 2 (47%)	Risk ranges from about 1 in 8 (13%) to about 1 in 2 (53%)	
Pre-eclampsia in future pregnancy	Risk ranges from 1 in 50 (2%) to about 1 in 14 (7%).	Risk up to about 1 in 6 (16%) No additional risk if interval before next pregnancy < 10 years	If birth was needed before 34 weeks risk is about 1 in 4 (25%) If birth was needed before 28 weeks risk is about 1 in 2 (55%)
Cardiovascular disease	Increased risk of hypertension and its complications	Increased risk of hypertension and its complications	Increased risk of hypertension and its complications
End-stage kidney disease		If no proteinuria and no hypertension at 6–8 week postnatal review, relative risk increased but absolute risk low. No follow-up needed	
Thrombophilia		Routine screening not needed	

Crucial to the syndrome of pre-eclampsia is impaired placentation with deficient remodelling of the spiral arteries in early pregnancy. As a result placental blood flow is reduced. In recent years two theories of pathogenesis have been described. The *two-stage* process proposes that intermittent perfusion of the intervillous space results in periods of hypoxia which cause factors to be released into the circulation. These factors damage the vascular endothelium triggering a multisystem disorder with protein and fluid leaking into the intravascular space. The *continuum* theory suggests that pre-eclampsia is an increased maternal immune response to trophoblastic debris. The abnormal response may be due to the presence of increased amounts of debris (owing to impaired placental perfusion or a large placenta) or normal amounts of debris but abnormal maternal susceptibility.

To explain the different presentations of hypertensive diseases in pregnancy, it is proposed that some women will tolerate the physiological adaptations to pregnancy even if placentation is abnormal while others fail to tolerate the adaptations to a greater or lesser degree and develop gestational hypertension or pre-eclampsia.

PREDICTION OF PRE-ECLAMPSIA

Predicting who will develop pre-eclampsia has exercised the minds of researchers for many years. A clinically useful predictive test should be reliable, valid and efficient when performed early in pregnancy. If such a test became available, maternal and fetal monitoring could be directed to women considered to be at high risk. Moreover, such women could be offered interventions with the aim of reducing risk or ameliorating the condition.

The simplest method of prediction is to identify risk factors from the clinical history (Table 4.3). Unfortunately such factors have a relatively low predictive value even in combination. More sophisticated methods include Doppler ultrasound assessment of the uteroplacental circulation and the measurement of angiogenic factors in the maternal circulation. A meta-analysis of 74 studies (79,547 women) found that elevated second-trimester uterine artery pulsatility index with notching predicted pre-eclampsia with a positive likelihood ratio of 21 among high-risk women and 7.5 among low-risk women.[12] The same meta-analysis found uterine artery Doppler to be more predictive when performed in the second trimester than in the first.

Pre-eclampsia is characterized by failure of normal trophoblastic invasion of spiral arteries. Angiogenic molecules regulate this vascular remodelling and have been found to be significantly abnormal several weeks before the onset of clinical signs and symptoms. Markers studied to date include vascular endothelial factors, soluble fms-like tyrosine kinase 1 and placental growth factors.

Table 4.3   Risk factors for pre-eclampsia
Family history of pre-eclampsia
Primigravida
Multiple pregnancy
Assisted conception
Previous pre-eclampsia/eclampsia/HELLP syndrome
Extremes of reproductive age
Obesity
Diabetes mellitus
Chronic kidney disease
Chronic hypertension
Systemic lupus erythematosus
Antiphospholipid syndrome

Research is ongoing, and it is likely that prediction of clinically important outcomes will require a combination of assessments, for example uterine artery Doppler, angiogenic markers and clinical history.

REDUCING THE RISK OF PRE-ECLAMPSIA

Administration of antiplatelet drugs in pregnancy is associated with a statistically significant reduction in the risk of pre-eclampsia for women considered at risk of the condition.[13] NICE 2010 guidance recommends that all women should have their risk of developing pre-eclampsia assessed early in pregnancy.[1] Those with one high risk factor or with more than one moderate risk factor (see below) should be offered 75 mg of aspirin daily from 12 weeks of pregnancy until the birth of their baby. It remains to be determined which women are most likely to benefit from this intervention, when treatment should start, and at what dose.

NICE (2010) risk factors:[1]

a. High risk factors
- hypertensive disease during a previous pregnancy
- chronic kidney disease
- autoimmune disease such as systemic lupus erythematosis or antiphospholipid syndrome
- type 1 or type 2 diabetes
- chronic hypertension

b. Moderate risk factors
- first pregnancy
- age $\geq$ 40 years
- pregnancy interval of more than 10 years
- BMI $\geq$ 35 at first visit
- family history of pre-eclampsia
- multiple pregnancy

Calcium supplementation is associated with a reduced risk of pre-eclampsia.[14] The benefit appears to be mainly for high-risk women and those with a low dietary intake of calcium. The optimum dose for supplementation has yet to be determined. Nutritional supplements, specifically folic acid, fish oils, and antioxidants such as vitamins C and E, have not been shown to reduce the risk of pre-eclampsia.

MANAGEMENT OF PRE-ECLAMPSIA

The majority of adverse maternal and perinatal outcomes from hypertension in pregnancy are due to pre-eclampsia/eclampsia/HELLP syndrome. Table 4.4 lists the complications of pre-eclampsia. Women with pre-eclampsia should be admitted to hospital for assessment of maternal and fetal condition. Subsequent

Table 4.4 Complications of pre-eclampsia

Maternal	Fetal/neonatal
Cerebral haemorrhage	Growth restriction
Eclampsia	Intrauterine fetal death
Pulmonary oedema	Prematurity (usually iatrogenic due to deteriorating maternal
Adult respiratory distress syndrome	condition)
Cortical blindness	
Renal failure	
Hepatic rupture	
HELLP syndrome	
Thromboembolism	
Disseminated intravascular coagulation	
Placental abruption	

management depends on the level of blood pressure, gestational age, and results of tests of maternal and fetal wellbeing.

Maternal monitoring and management of hypertension (NICE 2010)[1]

1. Pre-eclampsia with mild hypertension (blood pressure140/90–149/99 mmHg)
   - Antihypertensive medication is not required.
   - Blood pressure should be measured at least four times a day.
   - Repeat quantification of proteinuria is not necessary.*
   - Maternal renal and liver function and platelet count should be monitored twice a week using pregnancy-specific ranges.[15]

2. Pre-eclampsia with moderate hypertension (blood pressure150/100–159/109 mmHg)
   - Treat hypertension to keep diastolic blood pressure 80–100 mmHg and systolic blood pressure < 150 mmHg.
   - Oral labetalol is recommended as first-line antihypertensive medication.
   - Blood pressure should be measured at least four times a day.
   - Repeat quantification of proteinuria is not necessary.*
   - Maternal renal and liver function and platelet count should be monitored three times a week.

3. Pre-eclampsia with severe hypertension (blood pressure ≥ 160/110 mmHg)
   - Treat hypertension to keep diastolic blood pressure 80–100 mmHg and systolic blood pressure < 150 mmHg.
   - Oral labetalol is recommended as first-line antihypertensive medication.
   - Blood pressure should be measured more than four times a day, depending on clinical circumstances.

- Repeat quantification of proteinuria is not necessary.*
- Maternal renal and liver function and platelet count should be monitored three times a week.

* The amount of proteinuria is a poor predictor of complications in women with pre-eclampsia. Thus the quantification of proteinuria in women with pre-eclampsia does not need to be repeated after confirmation of significant proteinuria (urinary PCR > 30 mg/mmol or 24-hour urine collection > 300 mg).

Fetal monitoring

An individual plan for fetal monitoring should be made depending on gestation at diagnosis, severity of hypertension and any previous history of pre-eclampsia, stillbirth or a small-for-dates baby. Fetal cardiotocography, ultrasound assessment of fetal growth, amniotic fluid volume and umbilical artery Doppler velocimetry should be carried out at diagnosis. Ultrasound measurements should be repeated at a minimum of every two weeks. More frequent assessments of amniotic fluid volume and umbilical artery Doppler are indicated if the results are abnormal. Cardiotography should be repeated at least once a week and more often if there is any change in fetal movements, vaginal bleeding, abdominal pain or deterioration in maternal condition.

Timing of delivery

The indications for delivery in pre-eclampsia are shown in Table 4.5.

The aim is to reach at least 34 weeks gestation if maternal condition and fetal wellbeing remain satisfactory. If delivery is anticipated before 34 completed weeks, a course of corticosteroids should be administered to enhance fetal lung maturity. Timing of premature delivery will depend on the availability of a cot and, if none is available, in-utero transfer to another unit. After 37 weeks delivery should be advised, as there is no maternal or fetal benefit of prolonging pregnancy.

Management of delivery

When the decision has been made to deliver the fetus, the mode of delivery will depend on the gestation (usually caesarean section at less than 36 weeks of gestation), the severity of the disease and the presence or absence of any associated obstetric complication. If a vaginal delivery is attempted, the woman should be regarded as

---

Table 4.5 Pre-eclampsia: indications for delivery

Severe maternal hypertension refractory to treatment

Deteriorating maternal condition (renal impairment, abnormal liver function tests, thrombocytopenia)

Pulmonary oedema

Eclampsia

HELLP syndrome

Evidence of fetal compromise: static fetal growth and/or abnormal tests of fetal wellbeing (fetal heart rate abnormalities and/or abnormal umbilical artery Doppler and/or oligohydramnios)

---

high-risk and her fetus should be monitored continuously. Regional anaesthesia can be employed if the platelet count is greater than 80×10^9/L and is preferable to general anaesthesia if delivery is by caesarean. Endotracheal intubation is associated with a rise in blood pressure and may be difficult in pre-eclampsia due to laryngeal oedema.

Ergometrine/Syntometrine should be avoided for the third stage since it can produce an acute rise in blood pressure. Oxytocin alone is used for prophylaxis of postpartum haemorrhage in the third stage of labour or after caesarean section.

The management of the woman with severe pre-eclampsia should take place in appropriate surroundings, such as a high-dependency/intensive-therapy room on the labour ward. Care should be supervised by senior obstetricians, anaesthetists and paediatricians working to an agreed protocol including the use of maternal early-warning scores.

Haematological and biochemical investigations should be repeated regularly. Fluid balance and renal function must be closely monitored to prevent iatrogenic complications such as pulmonary oedema, left ventricular failure and adult respiratory distress syndrome. Pulmonary oedema may result both from the over-administration of intravenous fluids and also from the damage to the endothelium of the pulmonary vessels that occurs in pre-eclampsia. Intravenous fluids should be restricted to maintenance crystalloids (no more than 85 mL/hour, or urine output in preceding hour plus 30 mL) and urine volumes measured hourly from an indwelling urinary catheter.

Seizure prophylaxis

Once the benefits of magnesium sulphate for both acute control of seizures and prevention of recurrence was demonstrated (see *Eclampsia*, below), the question arose as to whether this drug could be used in pre-eclampsia to prevent eclampsia. The Magpie trial compared magnesium sulphate to placebo in the management of pre-eclampsia where there was clinical uncertainty about magnesium sulphate.[16] Eligible women were either pregnant or had delivered within 24 hours and had a blood pressure of 140/90 mmHg or greater and 1+ or more proteinuria. Administration of magnesium sulphate halved the risk of eclampsia, and there was a trend towards reduced risk of maternal death. In the short term, there did not appear to be any harmful maternal or neonatal effects. However, about 25% of women reported side effects such as flushing, nausea/vomiting, muscle weakness, headache and palpitations. The trial concluded that magnesium sulphate should be considered for women with pre-eclampsia for whom there is a concern about the risk of eclampsia. In practice there will be women with pre-eclampsia (antepartum or postpartum) and any of the following:

- severe hypertension (especially if difficult to control) and proteinuria
- mild or moderate hypertension and proteinuria with one or more of:
  - severe headache
  - persistent visual disturbance

- epigastric or right hypochondrial pain/liver tenderness
- signs of clonus (≥ 3 beats)
- vomiting
- papilloedema
- HELLP syndrome/AST or ALT rising above 70 iu/L
- platelet count $< 100 \times 10^9$/L

The regime for administering magnesium sulphate is a bolus dose of 4 g followed by a continuous infusion of 1 g per hour for 24 hours.

Postpartum care

Women with severe pre-eclampsia will require initial postpartum care in HDU/ITU.

Their condition may deteriorate in the 24–48 hours after birth and then start to improve. The frequency of blood pressure measurements will depend on the severity of hypertension (every 15–30 minutes if severe, at least four times a day if mild or moderate hypertension). Blood pressure level should be kept below 150/100 mmHg. Once the level is stable below 130/80 mmHg, antihypertensive treatment can be reduced. Be alert for new-onset hypertension in women with pre-eclampsia who did not require antihypertensive medication before birth. Treatment should be started if blood pressure is 150/100 mmHg or higher (see *Postpartum hypertension*, below).

Monitoring of haematological and biochemical parameters should continue until the results are normal. The frequency of testing will depend on the clinical condition and previous evidence of renal, hepatic or haematological dysfunction. Postpartum fluid input should be restricted to 80–90 mL per hour or urine output plus 30 mL, to minimize the risk of pulmonary oedema. It is common in severe disease, particularly after delivery, to have transient oliguria, which may last for 24 hours or more. Seizure prophylaxis with magnesium sulphate at 1 g/hour should be continued for a total of 24 hours. In the absence of a coagulopathy or obstetric bleeding women should receive a prophylactic dose of low-molecular-weight heparin and compression stockings to reduce the risk of venous thromboembolism.

Women can be discharged to community care once their blood pressure is stable below 150/100 mmHg and any renal, hepatic or haematological abnormalities have resolved or are resolving. A plan of care should be outlined including frequency of blood pressure monitoring and thresholds for reducing or stopping antihypertensive treatment. If a woman still requires antihypertensive treatment 2 weeks after transfer to community care then her management should be reviewed by her general practitioner.

Following pre-eclampsia/eclampsia/HELLP syndrome women should be offered a medical review 6–8 weeks postpartum. This is an opportunity to review blood pressure control, test for proteinuria, ensure haematological and biochemical parameters have returned to normal, and to discuss contraception and the implications for future pregnancies and long-term health (Table 4.2). Women requiring antihypertensive medication 6–8 weeks postpartum should be referred to a specialist for investigation. If proteinuria $\geq$ 1+ is present 6 weeks postpartum, a further review is recommended at 3 months. Persistent proteinuria at 3 months postpartum is an indication for referral to a renal physician.[1]

Eclampsia

Eclampsia is the occurrence of convulsions in pregnancy or postpartum, not due to a primary neurological problem, in a woman with signs and symptoms of pre-eclampsia. It is caused by cerebral involvement of the disease and is thought to involve vasospasm leading to ischaemia, disruption of the blood–brain barrier and cerebral oedema. Forty-four per cent of cases occur postnatally, 38% in the antepartum period and 18% intrapartum. In over one-third of women, it may be the first obvious manifestation of pre-eclampsia. Signs and symptoms which may precede eclampsia include headaches and visual disturbance, epigastric or right upper quadrant pain, nausea and vomiting, rapidly increasing swelling of face and legs. The neurological complications of eclampsia include coma, focal motor deficits and cortical blindness. Cerebral haemorrhage complicates 1–2% of cases.

MANAGEMENT

The immediate management of eclampsia requires maintaining oxygenation, and administering medication to control seizures, prevent recurrence and treat severe hypertension. If antepartum, the priority is to stabilize the woman. Only then should fetal wellbeing be assessed and a plan made for delivery. Eclampsia is an obstetric emergency, and all staff should be experienced in an eclampsia drill, an example of which is shown in Table 4.6. An eclampsia drug box containing the required number of vials of magnesium sulphate, antihypertensive medication and calcium gluconate should be available in all clinical areas.

Magnesium sulphate is the anticonvulsant of choice for the control of eclamptic seizures and prevention of recurrence. It has been compared to phenytoin and diazepam in randomized trials and shown to be superior in preventing recurrent seizures, maternal death and severe morbidity. Magnesium sulphate is a membrane stabilizer and a vasodilator and therefore reduces cerebral ischaemia and limits any associated neuronal damage. It may also act as a central anticonvulsant in the hippocampus.

Magnesium toxicity causes loss of deep tendon reflexes, followed by respiratory depression and ultimately respiratory arrest. In most cases it is not necessary to measure serum magnesium levels, and therapy can be monitored safely by hourly measurement of the patellar reflex, respiratory rate and oxygen saturation. Magnesium is excreted by the kidneys, so particular caution is required if renal function is impaired.

Table 4.6   Eclampsia drill

Get help

Emergency obstetric team (consultant obstetrician, registrar and SHO, senior anaesthetist, senior midwife)

Locate eclampsia box and crash trolley

Airway
- Ensure patency
- Left lateral position
- Oxygen via a mask
- Pulse oximeter

Breathing
- Assess and support

Circulation
- Blood pressure and pulse
- Intravenous access

Immediate management to control seizures
- Intravenous bolus of magnesium sulphate 4 g over 15 minutes

Secondary management to prevent further seizures and severe hypertension
- Magnesium sulphate infusion at 1 g/hour for 24 hours to prevent further seizures
- Measure blood pressure every 10–15 minutes
- Commence a labetalol infusion (or hydralazine if woman has asthma) if systolic > 150 mmHg or diastolic > 100 mmHg on two or more occasions

---

Magnesium sulphate **should be discontinued** if any of the following occur:
- patellar reflex absent
- respiratory rate < 14 per minute
- oxygen saturation < 95%
- impaired maternal renal function – either oliguria, i.e. < 20 mL urine output per hour (over a period of 3–4 hours), or rising urea and creatinine levels

If there is concern about respiratory depression administer 10 mL of 10% calcium gluconate intravenously *slowly* over 10 minutes.

Once maternal seizures have ceased and blood pressure is controlled, and the woman is undelivered, fetal wellbeing should be assessed and preparations made for delivery. If fetal monitoring is satisfactory, gestation is more than 34 weeks and the cervix is favourable, then induction of labour can be considered. Delivery by caesarean section is indicated if there are concerns about fetal wellbeing, or if induction is likely to be prolonged.

Complications of eclampsia include death (1–2%) and morbidity such as coma, focal deficit, cortical blindness and cerebrovascular accident. Posterior reversible encephalopathy syndrome (PRES) is a rare complication of eclampsia. The signs/symptoms of this condition – headache, seizure, confusion, visual loss – are

Table 4.7	Causes of convulsions during pregnancy and within 48 hours of birth

Eclampsia

Epilepsy

Metabolic causes (e.g. hypoglycaemia)

Intracerebral pathology (haemorrhage, cerebral vein thrombosis, ischaemic stroke)

Meningitis

Drug/alcohol-related

Cerebral hypoxia (hypotension, high sympathetic block)

Oxytocin-induced water intoxication

Hyperventilation

Thrombotic thrombocytopenia purpura/haemolytic uraemic syndrome

thought to be due to cerebral oedema. Although eclampsia is the commonest cause of seizures associated with pregnancy, other aetiologies should be considered (Table 4.7). Women with persistent neurological signs/symptoms require a CT/MRI scan and neurological review.

HELLP syndrome

Mild abnormalities of liver enzymes and platelet count are common in pre-eclampsia. HELLP syndrome (haemolysis, elevated liver enzymes and low platelets) affects up to 20% of women with severe pre-eclampsia and is associated with a high maternal and perinatal mortality and morbidity. The classic histological hepatic appearance of HELLP syndrome is periportal or focal parenchymal necrosis in which large hyaline deposits of fibrin-like material can be seen in the sinusoids.

HELLP syndrome may present antepartum or postpartum. The clinical features include:

- epigastric or right upper quadrant pain (65%)
- nausea and vomiting (35%)
- tenderness in right upper quadrant
- hypertension with or without proteinuria
- placental abruption (16%) – may be presenting feature
- haematuria
- jaundice

These signs and symptoms are not specific to HELLP, and the syndrome may be misdiagnosed, especially in its early stages. Hypertension and proteinuria may be absent.

LABORATORY DIAGNOSIS

- evidence of haemolysis on a peripheral blood smear, increased bilirubin and increased lactic dehydrogenase
- elevated liver transaminases > 70 iu/L
- low/falling platelet count, usually < 100 × 10^9/L

DIFFERENTIAL DIAGNOSIS

- thrombotic thrombocytopenic purpura
- haemolytic uraemic syndrome
- acute fatty liver of pregnancy

COMPLICATIONS OF HELLP

- abruption
- liver haematoma/rupture
- acute renal failure

MANAGEMENT

Care should follow the principles for severe pre-eclampsia. Women will require HDU/ITU care with careful monitoring of hepatic and renal function, platelet count and clotting profile. If HELLP develops antepartum, delivery is indicated once the maternal condition is stable. Antihypertensive medication may be required, and, if preterm, steroid therapy should be given to accelerate fetal lung maturity. The method of delivery will depend on the gestation, cervical ripeness and fetal wellbeing. Transfused platelets are rapidly consumed, so platelet transfusion is not beneficial unless caesarean section is required or there is active bleeding. Regional analgesia may be administered if platelet count is greater than 80 × 10^9/L.

Recovery from HELLP is usually spontaneous as long as the woman is delivered. However, the maternal condition may deteriorate in the immediate postpartum period. Until maternal condition stabilizes, HDU/ITU care should continue with use of maternal early-warning charts and close monitoring of blood pressure and fluid balance. The use of postpartum steroid therapy to accelerate normalization of blood parameters remains unproven.

In future pregnancies, women are at risk of developing pre-eclampsia (Tables 4.2, 4.3) but their risk of recurrent HELLP is less than 5%.

Postpartum hypertension[17]

In normotensive women, blood pressure normally falls for 24–48 hours after birth and then rises again, reaching a peak 3–6 days postpartum. About 12% of women will have a diastolic blood pressure greater than 100 mmHg in the first few days after delivery, which is thought to be due to normal postpartum fluid shifts.

AETIOLOGY OF HYPERTENSION IN THE POSTPARTUM

- Pre-existing hypertension, i.e. present before delivery. This may be chronic hypertension, pre-eclampsia/eclampsia or gestational hypertension.
- New-onset hypertension arising for the first time in the postpartum period
- Transient hypertension secondary to pain, anxiety, medications (e.g. ergometrine, non-steroidals), excess fluid administration and/or postpartum fluid shifts

Pre-eclampsia and gestational hypertension are the most common causes of post-partum hypertension. Retrospective studies suggest that 50–85% of women with pre-eclampsia or gestational hypertension will have a normal blood pressure by 7 days post-delivery. Factors associated with persistent hypertension include longer duration of antihypertensive treatment in pregnancy, high maximum blood pressures (> 160/100 mmHg), higher BMI and preterm pre-eclampsia.

The incidence of new-onset postpartum hypertension is unknown. There is no reliable method of early detection. The NICE 2010 guideline advises:[1]

- measuring BP within 6 hours of delivery for all uncomplicated pregnancies and on day 5 postpartum
- informing women of signs and symptoms which may indicate hypertension/pre-eclampsia, such as severe headache unrelieved by regular analgesia, visual disturbances, nausea. However, some of these symptoms are not specific for hypertension/pre-eclampsia

WHY DETECT AND TREAT POSTPARTUM HYPERTENSION?

The immediate clinical reason is to prevent complications of severe hypertension/pre-eclampsia, e.g. cerebral haemorrhage, eclampsia. In the longer term, if hypertension persists postpartum it may have a treatable underlying secondary cause such as adrenal disease.

ANTIHYPERTENSIVE TREATMENT

The blood pressure of women with pregnancy-related hypertension persisting postpartum often falls immediately postpartum, and medication may not be required for the first 12–24 hours. Once blood pressure reaches 150/100 mmHg or greater, antihypertensive medication should be commenced or increased. Options for treatments include labetalol, atenolol, calcium channel antagonists (drug of choice for black women of African or Caribbean origin) and the ACE inhibitor enalapril. Methyldopa should be avoided because of its association with depression.

Key summary points

- A multidisciplinary approach is fundamental to good management. Advice should be sought from obstetricians, anaesthetists, paediatricians and laboratory staff.
- Treatment should take account of the individual woman's needs and preferences.
- Good communication, supported by evidence-based information, is essential to enable women and the professionals caring for them to agree a plan of management.
- Senior staff (consultant obstetrician, labour ward coordinator, consultant anaesthetist and neonatal paediatrician) should be involved early in the assessment and management of any woman admitted with severe pre-eclampsia, eclampsia or HELLP syndrome.
- Maternal early-warning score charts should be used to monitor women admitted with hypertensive conditions.
- Hypertension > 150 mmHg systolic requires antihypertensive therapy.
- Be alert to the risk of fluid overload and pulmonary oedema in pre-eclampsia, eclampsia and HELLP syndrome.
- Women who have had a pregnancy complicated by pre-eclampsia are at risk of hypertension and cardiovascular disease in later life.

References

1. National Institute for Health and Care Excellence (NICE). *Hypertension in Pregnancy: the Management of Hypertensive Disorders during Pregnancy.* NICE Clinical Guideline CG107. London: NICE, 2010.

2. Knight M, Tuffnell D, Kenyon S, *et al.* (eds.) on behalf of MBRRACE-UK. *Saving Lives, Improving Mothers' Care: Surveillance of Maternal Deaths in the UK 2011–13 and Lessons Learned to Inform Maternity Care from the UK and Ireland Confidential Enquiries into Maternal Deaths and Morbidity 2009–13.* Oxford: National Perinatal Epidemiology Unit, 2015.

3. Knight M. Eclampsia in the United Kingdom 2005. *BJOG* 2007; 114: 1072–8.

4. Centre for Maternal and Child Enquiries (CMACE). *Perinatal Mortality 2009: United Kingdom.* London: CMACE, 2011.

5. Magee LA, von Dadelszen P, Rey E, *et al.* Less-tight versus tight control of hypertension in pregnancy. *N Engl J Med* 2015; 372: 407–17.

6. Walker JJ. Daycare assessment and hypertensive disorders of pregnancy. *Fetal Matern Med Rev* 1994; 6: 57–70.

7. Tuffnell DJ, Lilford RJ, Buchan PC, *et al.* Randomised controlled trial of day care for hypertension in pregnancy. *Lancet* 1992; 339: 224–7.

8. Twaddle S, Harper V. An economic evaluation of daycare in the management of hypertension in pregnancy *Br J Obstet Gynaecol* 1992; 99: 459–63.

9. Action on Pre-eclampsia. Pre-eclampsia community (PRECOG) guidelines. http://action-on-pre-eclampsia.org.uk/professional-area/precog (accessed 3 October 2015).

10. Vijgen SM, Koopmans CM, Opmeer BC, *et al.* An economic analysis of induction of labour and expectant monitoring in women with gestational hypertension or pre-eclampsia at term (HYPITAT trial). *BJOG* 2010; 117: 1577–85.

11. Smith RA, Kenny LC. Current thoughts on the pathogenesis of pre-eclampsia. *The Obstetrician & Gynaecologist* 2006; 8: 7–13.

12. Cnossen JS, Morris RK, ter Riet G, *et al.* Use of uterine artery Doppler ultrasonography to predict pre-eclampsia and intrauterine growth restriction: a systematic review and bivariable meta-analysis. *Can Med Assoc J* 2008; 178: 701–11. doi:10.1503/cmaj.070430.

13. Duley L, Henderson-Smart DJ, Meher S, King JF. Antiplatelet agents for preventing pre-eclampsia and its complications. *Cochrane Database Syst Rev* 2007; (2): CD004659.

14. Hofmeyr GJ, Lawrie TA, Atallah AN, Duley L. Calcium supplementation during pregnancy for preventing hypertensive disorders and related problems. *Cochrane Database Syst Rev* 2010; (8): CD001059.

15. Nelson-Piercy C. Normal laboratory values in pregnancy/non-pregnancy. In *Handbook of Obstetric Medicine*, 4th edn. London: Informa Healthcare, 2010; p. 273.

16. Altman D, Carroli G, Duley L, *et al.*; Magpie Trial Collaboration Group. Do women with pre-eclampsia, and their babies, benefit from magnesium sulphate? The Magpie Trial: a randomised placebo-controlled trial. *Lancet* 2002; 359: 1877–90.

17. Bramham K, Nelson-Piercy C, Brown MJ, Chappell LC. Postpartum management of hypertension. *BMJ* 2013; 346: f894.

5 Prematurity

Victoria Stern and Dilly Anumba

Introduction

Preterm birth is the leading cause of perinatal morbidity and mortality worldwide. In the UK, almost 8% of births occur before 37 weeks gestation, and the incidence of early delivery is increasing. Greater use of assisted reproductive technology and higher maternal age and body mass index (BMI) all contribute to this change.

Preterm birth may be spontaneous or iatrogenic (e.g. following induction of labour for pre-eclampsia). While it remains important to avoid expediting delivery unnecessarily, research is increasingly focused on the prediction and prevention of spontaneous preterm labour, which accounts for ~40% of early deliveries, with a further 25% occurring after preterm premature rupture of membranes (PPROM).

Approximately 5% of early deliveries occur at extremely preterm gestations (< 28 weeks), and the perinatal period is particularly hazardous for these babies. Although survival and complication rates improve with increasing gestational age, moderate to late preterm births (32–36 weeks) are still associated with significant, potentially lifelong, morbidity.

Pathogenesis

Preterm birth is a heterogeneous clinical problem. Variations in aetiology probably underlie the difficulty in finding a single effective predictive test or treatment. It has been suggested that it may be best to view preterm birth as a syndrome, with a common 'effector pathway' leading to delivery, but triggered by a wide range of different pathological conditions. Such triggers include uterine over-distension, infection within the reproductive tract, uteroplacental ischaemia and cervical weakness (Figure 5.1).

Infection plays a role in ~30–40% of spontaneous preterm births. The commonest route of infection is the ascent of pathogens, through the cervix, from the lower genital tract. Haematogenous spread via the placenta is also recognized (as

Antenatal Disorders for the MRCOG and Beyond, Second Edition, ed. Dilly Anumba and Shehnaaz Jivraj. Published by Cambridge University Press. © Cambridge University Press 2016.

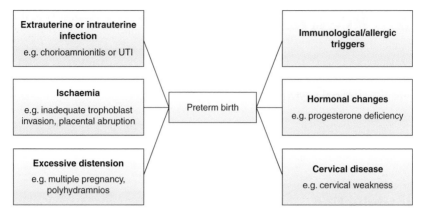

Figure 5.1 Pathological triggers of preterm birth. A black and white version of this figure will appear in some formats. For the colour version, please refer to the plate section.

illustrated by studies revealing colonization of the amniotic cavity with gingival microorganisms). Infection may be limited to the choriodecidual interface, or may spread across the membranes causing chorioamnionitis or even fetal infection (with a resultant fetal inflammatory response syndrome, FIRS). Microorganisms present within the uterus can stimulate contractions through the release of phospholipase A, which provokes local prostaglandin production. They also stimulate cervical ripening and weakening of the fetal membranes through the production of matrix metalloproteases/other proteolytic enzymes and heighten inflammatory mediator release (particularly interleukin-1 and tumour necrosis factor), which further drives prostaglandin production.

Over-distension of the uterus (as seen in multiple pregnancy, polyhydramnios or mullerian abnormalities) has been shown to induce increased expression of so-called 'contraction-associated proteins'. Such proteins include the oxytocin receptor, prostaglandin synthetic enzymes and receptors, and gap junction proteins (e.g. connexins) which facilitate propagation of action potentials and thus muscular contraction throughout the uterus.

Uteroplacental ischaemia (both chronic, as seen in intrauterine growth restriction, and acute, as seen in placental abruption) seems to provoke early labour. Observational studies have noted an increased incidence of abnormal vasculature in the placentas of preterm babies, such as failed transformation of the spiral arteries and thrombotic lesions. The mechanisms by which ischaemia precipitates labour are unclear, but stimulation of the local renin–angiotensin–aldosterone system or direct stimulation of uterine contractility by thrombin and hypoxia may play a role.

Cervical weakness is a well-recognized contributor to preterm birth. Women may have inherent problems with cervical function, or insufficiency may follow cervical surgery (particularly cone biopsy or multiple loop excisions). An overlap between infection-mediated preterm birth and cervical shortening has also become increasingly clear. Women with a short cervix have a much higher incidence of intrauterine infection. However, in practice it is unclear whether this finding is explained by reduced barrier function of the shortened cervix (which increases the risk of ascending infection) or by the reverse scenario, where intrauterine infection stimulates cervical ripening and shortening.

Understanding the causes and underlying pathways of preterm labour is key to developing effective tests and treatment, and knowledge in this area is continually developing.

Antenatal management

Strategies aiming to reduce the morbidity and mortality associated with preterm birth require the following steps:

- identification of women at increased risk of preterm birth
- provision of surveillance/screening tests
- administration of preventive treatments
- careful assessment and treatment of those presenting with threatened preterm labour

RISK ASSESSMENT

A multitude of factors have been associated with increased preterm birth (PTB) risk, some of which are modifiable, others not. Table 5.1 provides a summary of risk factors; this list is not exhaustive, but the presence of these features in a woman's history may be helpful in assessing and reducing her risk in future pregnancies.

A history of a previous preterm birth is the strongest historical predictor of early delivery. The recurrence rate for PTB in a singleton pregnancy following prior singleton PTB is ~20–25%. However, recurrence rates vary according to gestation of prior PTB (the earlier the gestation the higher the recurrence risk), number of prior preterm births and the occurrence of any term deliveries following the index PTB. Careful history taking is essential to assess the nature of the prior PTB and whether any non-recurrent triggers were present (e.g. traumatic abruption), to allow individualized counselling of patients.

Many of the other factors detailed above lack sensitivity in predicting preterm birth recurrence, but identifying modifiable risk factors will enable the woman to make changes to reduce her risk (including weight reduction, smoking cessation and modification of working patterns and life stressors). For healthcare providers, ensuring good access to antenatal care, particularly for vulnerable women, maximizing the availability of antenatal monitoring and avoiding iatrogenic multiple pregnancy (through cautious use of reproductive technologies) will all help reduce the preterm birth rate.

Table 5.1 Risk factors for preterm birth

Obstetric history	History of previous preterm birth/late miscarriage
	History of previous preterm premature rupture of membranes (PPROM)
	Prior obstetric cervical injury (e.g. tearing during vaginal delivery or second-stage caesarean section)
Maternal demographics	Extremes of maternal age
	Ethnicity (higher rates in non-white, particularly black, mothers)
	Socioeconomic status*
	Poor access to antenatal care*
Gynaecological history	Cervical treatment (especially previous cone biopsy/multiple loop excisions)
	Known bicornuate uterus/other mullerian abnormality
	Uterine septoplasty
Lifestyle factors	Smoking*
	Stress*
	Activity levels* (shift work/heavy physical labour associated with PTB)
	BMI*
	Short inter-pregnancy interval*
	Periodontitis*
Pregnancy-specific factors	Bleeding/antepartum haemorrhage
	Short cervix (< 25 mm before 24 weeks)
	Bacterial vaginosis (BV)
	Multiple pregnancy*
	Fertility treatment

* potentially modifiable factors

INVESTIGATIONS

Cervical length scanning

Ultrasound measurement of cervical length has an established role in preterm birth prediction. Although the cervix can be assessed by transabdominal and translabial routes, transvaginal ultrasound most sensitively identifies cervical shortening, is generally acceptable to women and has good reproducibility when performed by trained practitioners (Figure 5.2).

The technique for measuring cervical length is relatively simple:

- Ask the woman to empty her bladder.

- Gently introduce the covered transvaginal probe, while observing the image on screen and taking care not to compress the cervix excessively.

- Obtain a longitudinal section of the uterus and cervix, noting the presence of any funnelling or 'sludge' at the level of the internal os.

- Magnify the image to occupy two-thirds of the screen.

- Once a suitable image demonstrating the full length of the cervix has been obtained, withdraw the transducer slightly, enough to minimize application pressure to the cervix but maintain image quality.

(a)

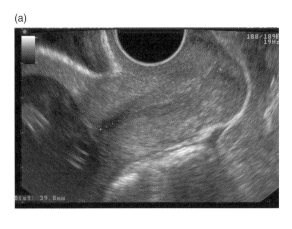

(b)

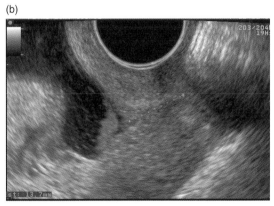

Figure 5.2 Transvaginal ultrasound illustrating (a) a normal cervical length and (b) a shortened cervix demonstrating funnelling. A black and white version of this figure will appear in some formats. For the colour version, please refer to the plate section.

- Place the calipers on the internal and external os and measure the cervical length (if the cervix is excessively curved a linear measurement may underestimate this).
- Repeat the measurement, obtaining three images with good reproducibility, and record the shortest obtained cervical length.

Several practice guidelines recommend that all women with a history of one or more prior preterm births or mid-trimester losses are offered serial cervical length scans, but acknowledge that expectant management may also be appropriate, as the majority of women with a history of preterm birth will go on to deliver after more than 33 weeks gestation. Screening regimes vary, but commonly scans are performed fortnightly, between 16 and 24 weeks. A cervical length $\geq$ 25 mm prior to 24 weeks is considered normal for women with a prior preterm birth, although thresholds for initiating treatment vary between studies.

It has been suggested that universal cervical length screening at the time of the anomaly scan might be utilized in the general obstetric population to identify those at high risk of preterm birth. This approach is not without problems: current evidence does not support the use of cervical cerclage in low-risk women with an incidental short cervix, and progesterone use in this group is also contentious. While it has been suggested by some that progesterone supplementation in women with cervical length < 15 mm may be of benefit, such treatment is unlicensed in the UK, and the Royal College of Obstetricians and Gynaecologists (RCOG) recommends restricting its use to clinical trials pending additional evidence. The limited positive predictive value of a short cervix in women without prior preterm birth is also a problem, with estimates ranging widely from 4% to 44%.[1]

Infection screening

An association between bacterial vaginosis (BV) and preterm birth has long been recognized. The most recent Cochrane review of antibiotic therapy for BV in pregnancy suggests that early screening and treatment can reduce the risk of late miscarriage (RR 0.2, 95% CI 0.05–0.76), but does not seem to reduce the rate of preterm birth < 37 weeks or PPROM.[2] Even when women with a prior history of preterm birth were considered, antibiotic treatment did not significantly reduce preterm birth rates. Other studies have suggested that gene–environment interactions may underlie the association between BV and early delivery: researchers have identified polymorphisms within several inflammation-regulating genes which, when present in association with BV, are associated with a particular increase in preterm birth risk. In future, if women with genetic susceptibility to the effects of BV can be identified reliably, they may be a group who demonstrate greater benefit from infection screening.

One large randomized study evaluated in a 2015 Cochrane review suggests that broader screening for lower genital tract infections (obtaining vaginal swabs for BV, candida and trichomonas and treating if positive) may reduce preterm birth (RR 0.55, 95% CI 0.41–0.75), although caregivers were not blinded to the woman's group assignment or screening results, and it was unclear if loss to follow-up was balanced between groups.[3]

Screening and treatment for asymptomatic bacteriuria in pregnancy has also been the subject of a systematic review. Its incidence varies from 2% to 10%, and treatment is known to reduce the risk of maternal pyelonephritis (RR 0.23, 95% CI 0.13–0.41). Although antibiotics did not seem to reduce the risk of preterm birth, a lower incidence of low fetal birth weight was noted in mothers receiving screening and treatment.

Periodontitis has also been associated with increased preterm birth rates in observational research. However, studies evaluating the effect of dental treatment on preterm birth rates have yet to show evidence of benefit.

Fetal fibronectin (FFN)

Fetal fibronectin is a glycoprotein which is normally present within the uterus, particularly at the interface between the decidua and membranes. It plays a role in adhesion of the membranes to the uterine wall, and disruption at this level (e.g. due to inflammation or membrane separation) can cause FFN to be released into the cervicovaginal discharge. In normal pregnancies, levels of FFN within the discharge should be low between 20 and 35 weeks gestation; if a high level is detected, this is associated with an increased risk of preterm birth. Current commercial testing kits require a swab to be obtained from the posterior vaginal fornix. This is then placed in a buffer solution and tested with a rapid bedside enzyme-linked immunosorbent assay (ELISA) which utilizes FDC-6 (a monoclonal antibody specific for FFN) to estimate FFN levels within the sample.

Many studies of FFN testing have focused on its use in women with symptoms of preterm labour (considered further below).[4] However, it is increasingly being used in the assessment of asymptomatic women at high risk of preterm birth. Testing may be qualitative ($<$ 50 ng/mL represents a negative FFN swab, $\geq$ 50 ng/mL is a positive result) or quantitative. The most clinically useful aspect of the test is its high negative predictive value (NPV): in asymptomatic high-risk women, NPVs of 86–98% have been reported, with higher NPV when predicting PTB over shorter time periods. Initial studies of quantitative FFN testing suggest improved positive predictive values (PPV): one series suggested a PPV of 62.5% for preterm birth $<$ 37 weeks when FFN levels of $\geq$ 200 ng/mL were detected in asymptomatic high-risk women. Practically speaking, a negative FFN swab in a patient at high risk of preterm birth may aid decision making (e.g. when deciding if admission is required when cervical shortening has been identified).

Other technologies

A multitude of other biomarkers and imaging techniques continue to be assessed in the hunt for better predictive tests. In a recent systematic review, 116 different serum or cervicovaginal biomarkers were identified but none has yet improved upon tests used in current clinical practice.[5] Cervical assessment has also been the focus of considerable work, with novel technologies (e.g. cervical elastography and fluoroscopy) aiming to quantify ripening changes within cervical stroma and the mechanical properties of the tissue in addition to measuring length alone. In future, successful screening may need to incorporate several of these tests, to allow a more comprehensive risk assessment.

In summary, the most successful screening approaches currently focus on monitoring women with a history suggestive of high preterm birth risk. Effective tests and interventions for low-risk populations have not yet been established. In women with risk factors for preterm birth, cervical length surveillance and early swabs for bacterial vaginosis may be offered. Quantitative fibronectin estimation may be offered via specialist clinics, and can aid clinical decision making.

PREVENTIVE TREATMENT

Cerclage

Cervical cerclage has been performed for over 100 years, but enthusiasm for the procedure has varied, as conflicting results of trials and meta-analyses have been published. It is unclear whether the inconsistent evidence of benefit in the literature results from inherent limitations of the procedure, or from difficulties selecting the patients who are most likely to benefit. Similarly, it can be difficult to evaluate which complications/side effects of cerclage result from treatment and which are due to underlying cervical incompetence/predisposition to infection. Its utility is further detailed in an RCOG guideline.[6]

Sutures can be inserted via transvaginal or transabdominal approaches. The transvaginal McDonald technique involves cerclage insertion just below the maternal bladder, and it can be removed without regional anaesthesia. The Shirodkar technique necessitates reflection of the bladder, enabling higher stitch placement, but as a result removal is more difficult. Transabdominal sutures may be placed using open or laparoscopic techniques, and are generally considered in those for whom transvaginal cerclage has failed, or after trachelectomy for neoplastic disease. Ongoing studies are addressing technique-specific questions; at present there are no recommendations regarding choice of suture material, placement of single versus double sutures, etc.

There are three scenarios in which cervical cerclage may be indicated:

- in a patient presenting with a history of prior PTB/mid-trimester loss (MTL) (**history-indicated cerclage**) – prophylactic insertion of a stitch in asymptomatic women at ~12–14 weeks

- in a patient with cervical length < 25 mm on transvaginal ultrasound scan (TVUSS) (**ultrasound-indicated cerclage**) – prophylactic insertion in asymptomatic women with a short cervix on TVUSS at 16–24 weeks

- in a patient presenting with premature cervical dilatation (**rescue cerclage**) – suture insertion once premature cervical dilatation has already commenced

History-indicated cerclage should be offered to women who have experienced three or more previous PTB/MTL. This recommendation is based on the results of a multicentre randomized controlled trial (RCT) which demonstrated a significant reduction in preterm birth rates after cerclage in this group (RR 0.47, $p < 0.05$), but only non-significant reductions in women with one or two prior PTB/MTL. Two smaller RCTs evaluating history-indicated cerclage in moderate- and high-risk women demonstrated no difference between intervention and control arms. Current UK guidance therefore advises that women with ≤ 2 prior PTB/MTL should be offered ultrasound surveillance of cervical length rather than history-indicated cerclage. A subsequent Cochrane review added weight to this conservative policy: meta-analysis of four studies (of 2045 women at high risk of PTB undergoing history-indicated cerclage or expectant management) showed a non-significant reduction in preterm birth < 37 weeks (RR 0.86, 95% CI 0.59–1.27), and similarly a non-significant reduction in perinatal loss (RR 0.8, 95% CI 0.58–1.1).[7] However, patient choice is an important factor in management decisions.

Two meta-analyses have evaluated the use of ultrasound-indicated cerclage versus expectant management in high-risk women with a short cervix. Berghella *et al.* observed significant reductions in preterm birth < 35 weeks when women with a prior PTB and cervical length < 25 mm were treated (RR 0.70, 95% CI 0.55–0.89).[8] They also noted a concurrent reduction in composite perinatal morbidity and mortality (RR 0.64, 95% CI 0.45–0.91). The 2012 Cochrane review by Alfirevic *et al.* similarly concluded that ultrasound-indicated cerclage can reduce preterm birth < 37 weeks (RR 0.55 [0.30, 0.99] for one-off and 0.78 [0.60, 1.02] for serial ultrasound-indicated cerclage) but did not demonstrate significant reductions in perinatal loss or morbidity.[7] UK guidance recommends offering ultrasound-indicated cerclage to high-risk women with cervical length ≤ 25 mm before 24 weeks, but not to women with isolated funnelling, or to low-risk women with an incidental short cervix.

The evidence base for rescue cerclage is very limited, with a few small studies suggesting insertion may delay delivery and reduce preterm birth. However, there is insufficient evidence to confirm whether these gestational gains translate into improved neonatal outcomes. Potential harm, particularly infectious morbidity for mother and neonate, have also not been adequately assessed. UK guidance therefore recommends individualized decision making by a senior obstetrician, with particular caution in cases presenting ≥ 24 weeks.

Progesterone

The use of antenatal progesterone prophylaxis is somewhat contentious. The literature evaluating its use is heterogeneous, with different populations studied (singleton vs. multiple pregnancies, previous history of preterm birth vs. no history), different outcome measures assessed and varying thresholds for therapy used. Unsurprisingly this has resulted in variation in international guidelines. The Royal College of Obstetricians and Gynaecologists (RCOG) currently advises that progesterone supplementation for the prevention of preterm birth should not be offered outside the context of a clinical research trial. This contrasts with guidelines in America, Canada and Australia, all of which recommend progesterone supplementation in specific circumstances.

Recent reviews of the evidence reveal a statistically significant reduction in preterm birth when progesterone is used in two patient groups: patients with a past history of spontaneous preterm birth (RR 0.31, 95% CI 0.14–0.69 for birth < 34 weeks; RR 0.55, 95% CI 0.42–0.74 for birth < 37 weeks) and patients with a short cervix diagnosed by transvaginal ultrasound (RR 0.64, 95% CI 0.45–0.90). The figures in brackets represent data from the most recent systematic review, which evaluated 36 RCTs including 8523 women.[9] In patients with a prior history of preterm birth, progesterone was also associated with significant reductions in perinatal mortality and morbidity, including the incidence of low birth weights at delivery, necrotizing enterocolitis and requirements for assisted ventilation. These reviews postdate both the UK and European guidelines, which both advise restricting progesterone use to clinical trials. The main concern for the study groups devising the RCOG and European Association of Perinatal Medicine (EAPM) guidelines was lack of safety data surrounding the use of progesterone, and also evidence regarding optimal timing, doses, formulation and route of progestogen therapy.[10,11] The 2013 update to the Cochrane review acknowledges that this remains an issue.

Specific safety concerns include the possibility of a higher rate of gestational diabetes in mothers treated with 17-alpha-hydroxyprogesterone-caproate (17-OHPC, a synthetic progestogen), higher rates of second-trimester miscarriage and stillbirth (a non-significant increase was noted in one placebo-controlled trial) and the potential for embryo toxicity. However, data regarding these concerns are conflicting and in general more safety questions have been raised regarding synthetic 17-OHPC than natural progesterone. As our understanding of the mechanisms by which both synthetic and natural forms work increases, study outcomes must continue to be carefully scrutinized to establish short- and long-term safety profiles for all forms of progestogen.

Cervical pessary

Cervical pessaries have been described as a treatment for cervical incompetence for over 50 years, but their use has only more recently been evaluated by randomized studies. Essentially, an appropriate-size silicone ring is fitted over the cervix, which compresses and supports the cervical canal. It has also been said to 'correct' forward angulation of the cervix – the shape of the pessary is such that it bends the cervix backwards slightly to face the posterior vaginal wall, which elongates it and may allow redistribution of pressure away from the cervix. However, at present the mechanism of action is not fully understood. A 2012 multicentre RCT evaluated the use of pessaries in women with a singleton pregnancy and cervical length < 25 mm and suggested that it significantly reduced the incidence of preterm birth < 34 and < 37 weeks when compared with expectant management (RR 0.24, 95% CI 0.13–0.43 for < 34 weeks; RR 0.36, 95% CI 0.27–0.49 for < 37 weeks).[12] A smaller single-centre RCT, in the same year, did not show significant reductions in PTB with pessary use, and at present further studies are ongoing. If these confirm benefit, then pessaries may in future offer an affordable treatment option to women with cervical shortening.

Bed rest

Cochrane reviews of bed rest to prevent preterm birth in women with both singleton and multiple pregnancies suggest no reduction in the incidence of preterm birth < 37 weeks (RR 0.92, 95% CI 0.62–1.37 for singletons; RR 0.99,

95% CI 0.86–1.13 for multiples), although there was a trend towards improved fetal growth in multiple pregnancies where bed rest occurred.[13] In view of this, bed rest should not be routinely advised for preterm birth prevention, although it is still utilized by clinicians in some individualized situations.

MULTIPLE PREGNANCY AND PRETERM BIRTH PROPHYLAXIS

It is important to note that so far prophylactic treatments have been considered for the prevention of singleton preterm birth. Unfortunately, when multiple pregnancies are considered, no effective prophylactic treatment has yet been identified. Neither intramuscular 17-OHPC nor vaginal progesterone decreases preterm birth rates in twin pregnancies. Cerclage insertion not only shows no benefit – in one trial it seemed to increase the risk of delivery < 35 weeks, although this was in a subgroup of only 39 women.

Symptomatic women

ASSESSMENT

Clinical diagnosis of preterm labour is notoriously unreliable. The majority of women presenting at preterm gestations with painful regular uterine contractions will not deliver during their admission, and indeed most will reach term. Careful assessment and judicious use of predictive tests will therefore avoid unnecessary admissions and treatment.

FETAL FIBRONECTIN

The background to FFN testing has been discussed above. Both qualitative and quantitative assays can be used in symptomatic women too: a negative FFN swab (threshold < 50 ng/mL) has high NPV for delivery within 14 days of testing (98%) and prior to 34 weeks (98%). Quantitative testing allows improved PPV in women with high fibronectin levels: a result of > 500 ng/mL has a PPV of 75% for delivery before 34 weeks.

ACTIM PARTUS

Actim Partus testing also involves the detection of cervicovaginal biomarkers, but it detects a different glycoprotein, phosphorylated insulin-like growth factor-binding protein. Test performance in symptomatic women is similar to FFN, with a 92% NPV for delivery within 14 days of testing. Actim Partus is cheaper than FFN and is not affected by the use of vaginal lubricants or recent intercourse (unlike FFN).

CERVICAL LENGTH SCANNING

In the UK cervical length scanning is used predominantly for screening asymptomatic women, but its role in the assessment of symptomatic women has been evaluated by multiple studies. These were summarized by a 2010 meta-analysis which suggested cervical lengths of 15 mm, 20 mm, and 25 mm are associated with NPVs of 94.8%, 96.3%, and 95.8%.[14] Other researchers suggest cervical length may allow stratification of risk in women with symptoms of preterm labour, identifying those who most require tocolytic treatment, or for whom FFN testing may be most helpful. Such combination, two-stage approaches to investigations and treatment may be associated with cost savings.

TREATMENT

Tocolysis

The idea of using medication to relax the uterus in preterm labour has inherent appeal. However, studies of tocolysis to date have not demonstrated overwhelming benefits of such an approach. Current RCOG guidance emphasizes the lack of evidence of long-term benefit from tocolytic medication: while certain drugs (nifedipine and atosiban) may delay delivery by up to 7 days, their use is not associated with a reduction in preterm birth, or in perinatal mortality or neonatal morbidity rates. It may therefore be appropriate not to use any tocolytic medication. They emphasize that women most likely to benefit from treatment are those at extremely preterm gestations and those requiring antenatal corticosteroids or in-utero transfer (see below), and in these groups tocolysis can be considered in order to 'buy time' for useful interventions proven to improve perinatal outcomes.

There are concerns that many of the older trials of tocolysis may have been limited by including women who were unlikely to benefit from treatment (e.g. those at late preterm gestations, or not truly in preterm labour), thus diluting estimates of their efficacy. However, many studies also lack long-term follow-up/safety data, so risks may also have been underestimated.

Comprehensive systematic reviews of each of the main classes of tocolytic have been conducted recently, since the publication of the RCOG guideline (see 2014 Cochrane reviews of calcium channel blockers; oxytocin receptor antagonists; betamimetics; nitric oxide donors; magnesium sulphate and combination tocolysis for preventing preterm birth). However, their findings are broadly in keeping with the above guidance.

Calcium channel blockers (mainly nifedipine) act by reducing calcium ion transfer into myometrial cells, interfering with actin and myosin binding and inducing smooth muscle relaxation. They reduce preterm birth within 48 hours compared to placebo/expectant treatment (RR 0.30, 95% CI 0.21–0.43) and appear to have some benefits over other tocolytics (betamimetics, oxytocin receptor antagonists and magnesium) with respect to prolonging pregnancy and reducing neonatal morbidity.[15] No effect on perinatal mortality was demonstrated.

Oxytocin receptor antagonists (ORAs) competitively block decidual and myometrial oxytocin receptors, reducing intracellular calcium release and prostaglandin production. Atosiban (the main ORA used clinically) is considerably more expensive than other tocolytics (particularly nifedipine). Meta-analysis of studies comparing ORA with placebo showed no reduction in birth within 48 hours (RR 1.05, 95% CI 0.15–7.43) or in perinatal mortality/morbidity. For the two studies directly comparing atosiban and nifedipine, no significant differences in delivery < 48 hours and preterm birth were demonstrated. Atosiban was associated with fewer maternal side effects.[16] In one study atosiban use was actually associated with an increase in extremely preterm birth, though methodological flaws may have confounded this result. As with other drugs, long-term safety data for ORAs is lacking.

There is currently no evidence to support the use of nitric oxide donors, magnesium sulphate or combinations of tocolytic drugs for preterm birth prevention.

Steroids

The benefits of antenatal corticosteroids are well established. Administration of intramuscular (IM) betamethasone or dexamethasone prior to preterm birth (between 24 weeks and 34 weeks 6 days) reduces the risk of respiratory distress syndrome, intraventricular haemorrhage, necrotizing enterocolitis and perinatal death. The most commonly used regimens are two 12 mg doses of betamethasone given 24 hours apart, or four 6 mg doses of dexamethasone given 12 hours apart. Side effects for a single course are minimal, though evidence from experimental work suggests that repeated courses of steroids are associated with a reduction in birth weight and potential detrimental effects on neurological development.

Benefits are maximal for delivery occurring between 24 hours and 7 days after administration. A single repeat course of steroids may be considered for women who received a first course at a very early gestation but present later with threatened preterm labour < 35 weeks. Growth-restricted babies may benefit from steroids given for preterm delivery up to 35 weeks 6 days.

In-utero transfer

Transfer to a unit with adequate facilities to care for the preterm neonate, should delivery occur, is associated with improved outcomes, and is more cost-effective than ex-utero transfer. Timely use of predictive testing, such as cervical ultrasound and FFN assessment, should minimize inappropriate transfers, and tocolytic cover may be useful to reduce the risks of travel.

Magnesium sulphate for fetal neuroprotection

The role of magnesium as a neuroprotective agent was raised by studies of women with pre-eclampsia. Children born to women given magnesium sulphate for seizure prevention were noted to have significantly lower rates of cerebral palsy. Further studies followed, and a 2009 systematic review demonstrated significant reductions in cerebral palsy with magnesium neuroprotection (RR 0.68, 95% CI 0.54–0.87). One small study raised concerns about drug safety, with a higher perinatal mortality rate in the neuroprotection arm, but a high proportion of deaths may have been coincidental (e.g. due to fetal anomalies or twin-to-twin transfusion), and subsequent meta-analyses have shown no effect on mortality rates. The RCOG Scientific Advisory Committee recommend considering its use for women in preterm labour, particularly at early gestations.[17]

Interestingly, school-age follow-up data have recently been published for two neuroprotection RCTs (of 500–700 women); both demonstrate no long-term differences in neurological disability. However, the authors acknowledge that by this stage many external factors may have influenced outcomes for these children, confounding the effects of the drug itself.

Management of women with PPROM

While many women who prematurely rupture their membranes will labour spontaneously, some will not. In this situation it is important to confirm the diagnosis of PPROM (generally by sterile speculum examination, though additional investigations may be helpful), exclude chorioamnionitis and make a careful plan for ongoing monitoring. An initial period of inpatient observation is helpful in assessing maternal and fetal wellbeing with regular observations and cardiotocography. Avoiding digital vaginal examination helps to prolong the latent period between PPROM and labour. If all remains well, then outpatient monitoring may be appropriate for some patients, with regular follow-up. Chorioamnionitis can be difficult to diagnose, and women should be advised to monitor their temperature regularly and report any symptoms of offensive vaginal loss, fever or abdominal pain.

Administration of oral erythromycin for 10 days after PPROM (250 mg orally four times daily) reduces the risk of chorioamnionitis, delivery within 48 hours and 7 days, neonatal infection and the risk of abnormal cerebral ultrasound results. These findings mainly result from the ORACLE studies, which notably did not show evidence of benefit when antibiotics were administered to women in preterm labour with intact membranes – indeed, infants born to those mothers had higher rates of cerebral palsy at 7 years of age, whereas those who had antibiotics for PPROM showed no long-term differences.[18] Administration of co-amoxiclav should be avoided because of an increased risk of necrotizing enterocolitis.

Current evidence does not support the use of tocolytics in women with PPROM, as there appears to be an increased risk of chorioamnionitits and neonatal infections, with no neonatal benefit.

Decisions regarding timing of induction of labour should be individualized depending on gestation at PPROM and the clinical situation. The RCOG recommends considering delivery from 34 weeks gestation, and ongoing studies are attempting to address whether expectant management or early induction is most beneficial in this patient group.

Perinatal issues

PARENTAL COUNSELLING

Careful counselling of women presenting with preterm labour is vital, given the risk of serious and potentially lifelong complications for preterm infants. Parents should ideally be seen by a senior obstetrician and neonatologist prior to delivery, to provide information about treatment of preterm labour, predicting outcomes for their baby, recommended intrapartum care, and what to expect at and after delivery, including issues surrounding resuscitation.

Data from the EPICure studies[19] may be helpful in counselling parents about fetal prognosis (Table 5.2), although these should ideally be complemented by local neonatal-unit data.

Management of women presenting with threatened preterm delivery between 23 weeks 0 days and 24 weeks 6 days is particularly challenging, as, even with optimal perinatal care, survival rates are low and disability rates high. There is international consensus that fetuses born at 22 weeks have not yet reached viability, and also agreement that after 25 weeks, active management is likely to be appropriate. For the 'grey area' between these gestation limits, individual factors such as estimated fetal weight, condition at the time of delivery and parental preferences should be considered when making resuscitation decisions. The RCOG's Scientific Impact paper *Perinatal Management of Pregnant Women at the Threshold of Infant Viability* provides useful additional information to inform these difficult clinical situations.[20] Plans for neonatal care will inform obstetric decision making, and the above guidance describes three possible management approaches: Active management, where fetal monitoring (+/- caesarean delivery if required) and full resuscitation are planned; passive management, where caesarean delivery would not be considered but resuscitation would be attempted; and palliative management, where comfort care is provided if a live birth occurs.

Table 5.2 EPICure 2 figures: rates of survival and survival without disability at extremely preterm gestations

Gestational age	22 weeks	23 weeks	24 weeks	25 weeks	26 weeks
Survival from onset of labour	1%	15%	36%	62%	75%
Survival of admissions to NICU	16%	29%	46%	69%	78%
Survival without disability from onset of labour	0.4%	8%	22%	43%	59%
Survival without disability of admissions to NICU	5%	14%	28%	47%	61%

MODE OF DELIVERY

A 2013 Cochrane review evaluating the risks and benefits of caesarean delivery for women in spontaneous preterm labour showed no advantage in terms of perinatal death rates (RR 0.29, 95% CI 0.07–1.14; three trials, 89 women) or birth injuries, but revealed an increase in major maternal complications (RR 7.21, 95% CI 1.37–38.08; four trials, 116 women).[21] Current evidence therefore does not support a policy of caesarean delivery to avoid intrapartum fetal stress/injury. The review only includes four studies of 116 women, however, and the authors emphasize that all studies were stopped early due to poor recruitment. Thus their findings should be interpreted with caution. Similarly, evidence of benefit from caesarean delivery with preterm breech presentation is sparse and conflicting.

In practice, preterm labour can be rapid, so making decisions about mode of delivery can be complicated by difficulty in accurately diagnosing the onset of labour. General principles for care of preterm babies intrapartum include: keeping the membranes intact as long as possible (which may protect against the mechanical stresses of labour); being alert to the higher chance of cord prolapse/malpresentation and performing examinations/scans promptly to diagnose this; avoiding fetal blood sampling and ventouse delivery in gestations < 34 weeks. If there is a history of PPROM in a woman in preterm labour, the use of intravenous antibiotics to reduce the risk of neonatal Group B *Streptococcus* infection should be considered.

Key summary points

- Preterm birth remains the principal cause of perinatal mortality and morbidity worldwide.
- Although neonatal survival of premature babies is improving, there has been little or no change in the prevalence of preterm birth.
- Prediction and prevention remain limited, the best tools for screening asymptomatic high-risk women being ultrasound assessment of cervical length and cervicovaginal secretions for fetal fibronectin among other compounds.
- Management of women in a subsequent pregnancy hinges on careful assessment of risk of recurrence, identifying those women who may benefit from progesterone therapy or cervical cerclage, treating any predisposing factors amenable to therapy, and optimizing care in a facility with the appropriate neonatal care facilities, liaising with paediatricians at all times.
- Women at high risk of premature delivery should be considered to receive steroids to aid fetal lung maturation.

References

1. Society of Obstetricians and Gynaecologists of Canada. Clinical Practice Guideline No. 257, Ultrasonographic Cervical Length Assessment in Predicting Preterm Birth in Singleton Pregnancies. *J Obstet Gynaecol Can* 2011; 33: 486–99.

2. Brocklehurst P, Gordon A, Heatley E, Milan SJ. Antibiotics for treating bacterial vaginosis in pregnancy. *Cochrane Database Syst Rev* 2013; (1): CD000262.

3. Sangkomkamhang US, Lumbiganon P, Prasertcharoensuk W, Laopaiboon M. Antenatal lower genital tract infection screening and treatment programs for preventing preterm delivery. *Cochrane Database Syst Rev* 2015; (5): CD006178.

4. Deshpande SN, van Asselt AD, Tomini F, *et al.* Rapid fetal fibronectin testing to predict preterm birth in women with symptoms of premature labour: a systematic review and cost analysis. *Health Technol Assess* 2013; 17: 1–138.

5. Menon R, Torloni MR, Voltolini C, *et al.* Biomarkers of spontaneous preterm birth: an overview of the literature in the last four decades. *Reprod Sci* 2011; 18: 1046–70.

6. Royal College of Obstetricians and Gynaecologists. *Cervical Cerclage.* Green-top Guideline No. 60. London: RCOG, 2011.

7. Alfirevic Z, Stampalija T, Roberts D, Jorgensen AL. Cervical stitch (cerclage) for preventing preterm birth in singleton pregnancy. *Cochrane Database Syst Rev* 2012; (4): CD008991.

8. Berghella V, Rafael TJ, Szychowski JM, Rust OA, Owen J. Cerclage for short cervix on ultrasonography in women with singleton gestations and previous preterm birth: a meta-analysis. *Obstet Gynecol* 2011; 117: 663–71.

9. Dodd J, Jones L, Flenady V, Cincotta R, Crowther C. Prenatal administration of progesterone for preventing preterm birth in women considered to be at risk of preterm birth. *Cochrane Database Syst Rev* 2013; (7): CD004947.

10. Di Renzo GC, Roura LC, Facchinetti F, *et al.* Guidelines for the management of spontaneous preterm labor: identification of spontaneous preterm labor, diagnosis of preterm premature rupture of membranes, and preventive tools for preterm birth. *J Matern Fetal Neonatal Med* 2011; 24: 659–67.

11. Royal College of Obstetricians and Gynaecologists. *The Use of Progesterone to Prevent Preterm Delivery.* 2010. https://www.rcog.org.uk/en/guidelines-research-services/guidelines/the-use-of-progesterone-to-prevent-preterm-delivery (accessed 28 July 2015).

12. Goya M, Pratcorona L, Merced C, *et al.*; Pesario Cervical para Evitar Prematuridad (PECEP) Trial Group. Cervical pessary in pregnant women with a short cervix (PECEP): an open-label randomised controlled trial. *Lancet* 2012; 379: 1800–6.

13. Sosa CG, Althabe F, Belizan JM, Bergel E. Bed rest in singleton pregnancies for preventing preterm birth. *Cochrane Database Syst Rev* 2015; (3): CD003581.

14. Sotiriadis A, Papatheodorou S, Kavvadias A, Makrydimas G. Transvaginal cervical length measurement for prediction of preterm birth in women with threatened preterm labor: a meta-analysis. *Ultrasound Obstet Gynecol* 2010; 35: 54–64.

15. Flenady V, Wojcieszek AM, Papatsonis DN, *et al.* Calcium channel blockers for inhibiting preterm labour and birth. *Cochrane Database Syst Rev* 2014; (6): CD002255.

16. Flenady V, Reinebrant HE, Liley HG, Tambimuttu EG, Papatsonis DN. Oxytocin receptor antagonists for inhibiting preterm labour. *Cochrane Database Syst Rev* 2014; (6): CD004452.

17. Royal College of Obstetricians and Gynaecologists. *Magnesium Sulphate to Prevent Cerebral Palsy Following Preterm Birth.* Scientific Impact Paper No. 29. London: RCOG, 2011.

18. Kenyon SL, Taylor DJ, Tarnow-Mordi W; ORACLE Collaborative Group. Broad-spectrum antibiotics for preterm, prelabour rupture of fetal membranes: the ORACLE I randomised trial. *Lancet* 2001; 357: 979–88.

19. Moore T, Hennessy EM, Myles J, *et al.* Neurological and developmental outcome in extremely preterm children born in England in 1995 and 2006: the EPICure studies. *BMJ* 2012; 345: e7961.

20. Royal College of Obstetricians and Gynaecologists. *Perinatal Management of Pregnant Women at the Threshold of Infant Viability: the Obstetric Perspective.* Scientific Impact Paper No. 41. London: RCOG, 2014.

21. Alfirevic Z, Milan SJ, Livio S. Caesarean section versus vaginal delivery for preterm birth in singletons. *Cochrane Database Syst Rev* 2013; (9): CD000078.

Further reading

RCOG Green-top Guidelines

Royal College of Obstetricians and Gynaecologists. *Cervical Cerclage.* Green-top Guideline No. 60. London: RCOG, May 2011.

Royal College of Obstetricians and Gynaecologists. *Tocolysis for Women in Preterm Labour.* Green-top Guideline No. 1b. London: RCOG, February 2011.

Royal College of Obstetricians and Gynaecologists. *Preterm Prelabour Rupture of Membranes.* Green-top Guideline No. 44. London: RCOG, October 2010.

Royal College of Obstetricians and Gynaecologists. *Antenatal Corticosteroids to Reduce Neonatal Morbidity.* Green-top Guideline No. 7. London: RCOG, October 2010.

RCOG Scientific Impact Papers

Royal College of Obstetricians and Gynaecologists. *Magnesium Sulphate to Prevent Cerebral Palsy Following Preterm Birth.* Scientific Impact Paper No. 29. London: RCOG, September 2011.

Royal College of Obstetricians and Gynaecologists. *Obstetric Impact of Treatment for Cervical Intraepithelial Neoplasia.* Scientific Impact Paper No. 21. London: RCOG, June 2010.

Royal College of Obstetricians and Gynaecologists. *Perinatal Management of Pregnant Women at the Threshold of Infant Viability: the Obstetric Perspective.* Scientific Impact Paper No. 41. London: RCOG, February 2014.

Royal College of Obstetricians and Gynaecologists. *Preterm Labour, Antibiotics and Cerebral Palsy.* Scientific Impact Paper No. 33. London: RCOG, February 2013.

NICE guidance

National Institute for Health and Care Excellence (NICE). *Preterm Labour and Birth.* NICE Guideline NG 25. London: NICE, November 2015.

6 Previous caesarean section

Madeleine MacDonald

Introduction

Previous caesarean delivery is one of the most common reasons for a multiparous woman to book under the care of a consultant in a successive pregnancy. It is therefore crucial for all clinicians working in antenatal clinics to understand the issues surrounding the antenatal care of women with a previous caesarean section and birth after a previous section.

Over the last three decades the rate of caesarean section globally has significantly increased; in England over a 15-year period the rate has doubled to around 24%,[1] and in the United States caesarean delivery now accounts for almost a third of all births.[2] Despite this increase, improvement in the outcome for neonates has not been shown. In England, there is wide variation in the rate of caesarean sections between delivery units (15% to greater than 30%), which cannot be completely explained by differences in demographics or caseloads.[1]

The overall rise in caesarean deliveries is multifactorial, with suggested reasons including:[2]

- historical ('one caesarean, always a caesarean')
- maternal preference/choice
- clinician's preference
- patient factors such as increasing maternal age and obesity
- changes in obstetric practice, e.g. the management of breech presentation
- availability of external cephalic version (ECV)
- training issues, such as a reduction in the levels of experience of clinicians working on labour wards or fewer rotational forceps deliveries
- failure to follow guidelines
- use of cardiotocographs
- increasing litigation

Antenatal Disorders for the MRCOG and Beyond, Second Edition, ed. Dilly Anumba and Shehnaaz Jivraj. Published by Cambridge University Press. © Cambridge University Press 2016.

This rapid rise in the rates of caesarean deliveries has led the World Health Organization (WHO) to develop guidelines on optimal caesarean delivery rate (10–15%), and a 'toolkit' to aid clinicians in reducing the rate of sections.[1] In England, the NHS Institute for Innovation and Improvement suggested that a caesarean section rate of less than 20% reflects best practice in antenatal and intrapartum care.[1]

Antenatal care for a woman who has had a previous caesarean delivery

The rationale for booking a pregnant woman who has had a previous caesarean section under a consultant is because of the recognized potential problems that can occur in a pregnancy after a previous section, such as the increased risk of placenta praevia and accreta and the risks associated with delivery, whether vaginal birth or repeat section.[3]

At the first visit to the antenatal clinic it is important to establish details from previous pregnancies and deliveries that may impact on the recommendation for mode of delivery in this pregnancy (Table 6.1), and in particular previous:

- pre-eclampsia
- breech presentation and mode of delivery
- preterm deliveries, including mode of delivery
- vaginal births prior to or after the caesarean delivery

The details of the previous caesarean section, especially the indication and type of incision made, should be reviewed.[2,3]

Table 6.1   A summary of the information required to make an informed decision regarding mode of delivery after a previous caesarean section

Previous pregnancy/ labour details	Previous caesarean section details	Potential problems arising in this pregnancy	Maternal considerations
Previous vaginal deliveries	Indication	Placenta praevia or accreta	Mother preference
Laboured spontaneously in the past	Dilatation at which it took place	Condition requiring likely induction of labour, e.g. gestational diabetes	Motivation for a particular mode of delivery
Pre-eclampsia	Operative notes – any extensions or incisions such as J or T	Multiple pregnancy	Future fertility plans/plans for size of family
Fetal macrosomia	Inter-pregnancy interval	Fetal macrosomia	Attitude towards risk
	Gestation at which caesarean section took place	Pre-eclampsia	

This information aids the clinician in counselling the woman about her individual risks associated with either trial of vaginal birth after caesarean section (VBAC) or planned elective lower-segment caesarean section (LSCS). All necessary information may not be immediately available at the first visit; however, the clinician should make reasonable efforts to obtain it, such as writing to the unit where the previous section took place if elsewhere.[3]

It is also essential to take into account the woman's own preferences, her plans for future pregnancies, her perception of risk and her motivation for a particular type of birth.[3,4] Recommendation or advice on future deliveries after the caesarean section may have been made immediately after the previous section, and it can be helpful to ask whether the woman remembers any such discussion or advice being given.

Although the counselling process should begin early in the woman's pregnancy, ideally in the first trimester, definite plans may need to be delayed until the third trimester. Factors that alter the recommended mode of delivery can develop after the booking visit: for example, whether the current pregnancy is singleton or multiple, the location of the placenta in relation to the previous scar, because of the increased risk of placenta praevia and accreta with a scarred uterus,[3] and development of conditions such as pre-eclampsia or gestational diabetes that may require early delivery or potential induction of labour. Pre-eclampsia is also associated with a reduction in the success of VBAC.[3]

Many units offer women a more detailed discussion of birth after caesarean section with specialist midwives in the form of individual counselling or group workshops ('VBAC workshops'). This may also provide an opportunity for the woman and her partner to explore any concerns they have regarding the future birth in a more informal environment, and it can help them to make a decision they feel most comfortable with.

The final decision is usually made in the third trimester at the antenatal clinic by the woman and her clinician. This should be clearly documented in the notes: both her handheld and the hospital notes. There also needs to be an agreed and documented plan should she go into labour or rupture her membranes prior to the date of any planned caesarean section, a plan for any induction if necessary and how an induction would be undertaken, and whether prostaglandins may be used or not.[4]

MORBIDLY ADHERENT PLACENTA

Placenta praevia appears to be more common after a caesarean section.[3] If identified on ultrasound scan at 20 weeks, especially if the placenta is anterior, a repeat scan for placental localization should be arranged at 32 weeks. This leaves enough time for further investigations such as a Doppler ultrasound or MRI scan (depending on the unit's guidelines and experience of the local radiologists) to be performed if the placenta remains anterior and low-lying, to exclude or identify a placenta accreta or percreta and put in place the necessary arrangements for delivery, for example involvement of interventional radiologists or urologists.

Options for birth after previous caesarean section

Two options for delivery exist for women who have had a previous caesarean section:

- trial of vaginal birth
- planned (elective) repeat caesarean section

A Cochrane review first published in 2004 and updated in 2013 concluded that at present each option has its own risks and benefits, and the evidence available to aid women and those caring for them in future pregnancies is from non-randomized sources that may be subject to bias.[5] This can lead to problems in counselling women, with the advice based on suboptimal evidence.

Some authors argue that comparing the outcomes of VBAC or repeat emergency caesarean section after a trial of labour with those after planned elective section is inappropriate, because most complications in the trial of labour group occur in the women whose VBAC is unsuccessful.[2]

When discussing risks associated with either option, it is important to consider the woman's understanding and attitude towards risk.[4] Clinicians should also ensure when counselling these women that their own preferences and perception of risk do not bias or 'lead' the patient into making a choice that she may not feel comfortable with.

Vaginal birth after caesarean section (VBAC)

Historically, women who were delivered by caesarean section were told that all future deliveries also needed to be by caesarean section.[2] However, medical opinion began to change in the 1970s and vaginal birth after caesarean section (VBAC) started to be offered to selected women. More recently reports of complications, such as uterine rupture associated with VBAC, led to a rise again in repeat section.[2] Today, after extensive reviews of the available evidence by bodies such as the Royal College of Obstetricians and Gynaecologists (RCOG),[3] the American College of Obstetricians and Gynecologists (ACOG),[2] the National Institute for Health and Care Excellence (NICE)[4] and the Cochrane Collaboration,[5] and the drive by the WHO to try to reduce rates of caesarean section worldwide,[1] VBAC has again become a safe choice for many women who have had one or two previous caesarean sections.

Overall success rate for VBAC quoted by the RCOG, NICE and ACOG is between 60% and 90%, with multiple factors significantly influencing an individual's chance of success (Table 6.2).[2–4]

Table 6.2 Factors that influence the chances of a successful VBAC[3,4]

Factors for successful VBAC	Factors against successful VBAC
Previous vaginal birth (87–90% chance of successful VBAC)	Previous caesarean section(s) indication was for labour dystocia
Spontaneous labour	Increased maternal age
Indication for previous caesarean was elective for breech presentation	Non-white ethnicity
	No previous vaginal birth
	Over 40 weeks gestation
	Maternal obesity
	Short stature
	Male infant
	Pre-eclampsia
	Short inter-pregnancy interval (< 2 years)
	Neonatal macrosomia (> 4000 g)
	Augmented or induced labour
	Previous caesarean section performed at a preterm gestation
	No epidural analgesia during labour

Although the Cochrane review identified no level 1 evidence to guide clinicians and women when making decisions regarding mode of delivery after previous caesarean section,[5] attempts have been made to devise decision-making aids using scoring systems to quantify the individual probability of a successful VBAC.[2,4] These systems use factors such as those in Table 6.2 to give a percentage chance of successful outcome for VBAC, and were developed from observational data on the outcomes of deliveries after previous caesarean sections. There is also some evidence, from a further observational study using one of these scoring systems, that women with less than a 60% chance of a successful VBAC have a higher rate of morbidity than those undergoing a planned elective section.[2]

CONTRAINDICATIONS TO VBAC

Women who have previously had a classical caesarean section should be advised that it is recommended they have a repeat elective caesarean section due to the higher risk of uterine rupture (2–9%) if the incision was a high vertical incision along the complete length of the body of the uterus. The risk of rupture for low vertical incisions and those who have had 'J-shaped' or 'inverted T' incision in the lower segment also have a higher risk of rupture of approximately 2%.[3]

Myomectomy and other complex uterine surgery may also lead to higher rates of uterine rupture, although data regarding the specific risks are lacking.[3] Advice should be sought if possible from the surgeon who performed the uterine surgery.

RISKS OF VBAC VERSUS ELECTIVE LSCS

The RCOG recommends that women should be informed antenatally about the risks of VBAC and planned elective LSCS, as shown in Table 6.3.[3]

There is no statistically significant difference in the rate of hysterectomy, venous thromboembolism or maternal death between VBAC and planned LSCS. However, the majority of the morbidity associated with VBAC occurs when it is unsuccessful and an emergency LSCS is required.[2] In these cases there is a significantly increased risk of uterine rupture, scar dehiscence, hysterectomy, blood transfusion and endometritis.[2,3]

When considering the risks associated with uterine rupture, it should be noted that there are significant discrepancies in the literature regarding the definition of uterine rupture and uterine scar dehiscence, which leads to difficulties in comparing rates of rupture between studies.[5] Some studies did not differentiate between asymptomatic scar dehiscence and catastrophic uterine rupture, whereas others only included cases where a catastrophic rupture had taken place.[5]

There is limited information regarding the risks associated with VBAC for women who have had two previous LSCS. However, the data suggest the risk of uterine rupture is not significantly different from women with one section,[2] although the rates of blood transfusion and hysterectomy appear to be greater.[3] Overall the chances of successful VBAC after one or two LSCS appears to be similar, and therefore VBAC is a possible option for some women who have had two LSCS.[2] Careful discussion regarding the paucity of good-quality evidence should take place, and a decision for VBAC in these women should be made with the involvement of a senior clinician. The operative notes of the second section should be reviewed to assess for any evidence of a particularly thin lower segment, extensions in the uterine wound at section, dense adhesions, bladder damage or suspected scar dehiscence. Any suggestion of such problems should prompt the clinician to advise against VBAC.

Table 6.3   Risks of VBAC and planned elective LSCS

Complication	Level of risk for planned VBAC	Level of risk for planned LSCS
Uterine rupture	0.22–0.74%	0
Blood transfusion	1.7%	1%
Endometritis	2.89%	1.8%
Perinatal mortality*	0.24%	0.093%
Intrapartum HIE	0.078%	0
Neonatal respiratory morbidity	2–3%	3–4%

* The increase in perinatal mortality for VBAC is thought to be mainly due to the increased rate of stillbirth after 37 weeks.

Planned repeat caesarean section

In choosing a repeat LSCS, consideration should be given to the woman's plans for family size, as the risk of morbidly adherent placenta, accreta or percreta, increases for each additional section. For accreta the risk after a second section is 0.31%, rising to 3.49% after five sections. This risk is further increased if placenta praevia is also present: 11% after two sections up to 67% after five. The risk of hysterectomy, bladder injury and blood transfusion also increases significantly for each additional section a woman undergoes.[3]

Currently, elective caesarean sections are usually recommended to be undertaken from 39 weeks gestation to reduce the risk of neonatal respiratory problems (transient tachypnoea of the newborn and respiratory distress syndrome[3]) although a recent small randomized controlled trial (RCT) has suggested that the risk of respiratory problems in neonates delivered by elective LSCS before 39 weeks may have been overestimated in previous studies.[6] At present it is also recommended that if an elective caesarean section is performed before 39 weeks, steroids for fetal lung maturity should be given.[3]

If a woman choses a repeat caesarean, a plan should be made in case labour starts before the planned section date. This should be documented in the notes and confirmed if the event occurs. Women should be made aware of the potential additional risks of performing a repeat LSCS in advanced labour, especially if there are no concerns for fetal wellbeing or uterine rupture, and that if she were to attend the labour suite already in advanced labour, the safest option might be to continue with the VBAC instead of reverting to planned caesarean section.[3]

Figure 6.1 shows a care algorithm for the antenatal care of women with a previous caesarean section.

Special circumstances

PRETERM DELIVERY

Women with a previous LSCS who are at higher risk of preterm labour should be made aware that there is no significant difference in the risks associated with VBAC and the chances of success if labour occurs before 37 weeks, and in fact the risk of uterine rupture may be lower than with VBAC at term.[3] From the available evidence there also appears to be no difference between preterm VBAC and elective repeat LSCS in terms of neonatal outcome.[3]

MULTIPLE PREGNANCY

In women with twins, no difference in the outcome of VBAC has been found when compared to women with singleton pregnancies.[2] Both maternal and neonatal risks associated with VBAC are no more likely to occur with twin gestations,[2] and therefore it is possible for a woman with twins to undergo trial of labour after a

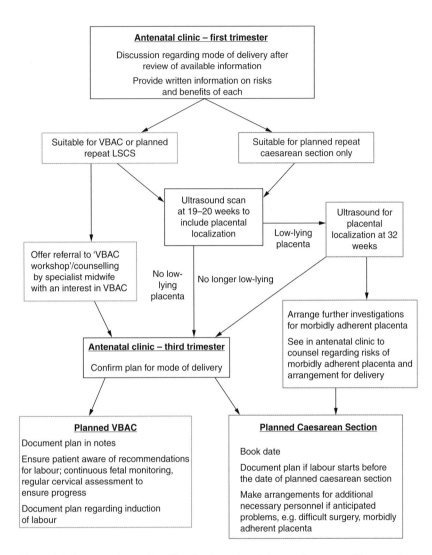

Figure 6.1 Suggested care algorithm for the antenatal care of women with a previous caesarean section. A black and white version of this figure will appear in some formats. For the colour version, please refer to the plate section.

previous caesarean section, especially if labour occurs spontaneously or if she has had a previous vaginal birth.

INDUCTION AND AUGMENTATION OF LABOUR

As previously alluded to, the chances of successful VBAC are significantly lower if labour is induced.[2,3] A woman with a previous LSCS for dystocia, who has never had a vaginal birth and has a BMI above 30, has only an estimated 40% chance of successful VBAC if induced.[3] Given that morbidity from unsuccessful VBAC is significantly greater than from planned repeat LSCS, if the chances of successful VBAC are less than 60%, planning induction of labour in these women should be considered very carefully.[2]

Induction or augmentation of labour carries a significantly increased risk of uterine rupture.[3] Data from the RCOG Green-top Guideline for VBAC suggests a 2–3-fold increase in rupture and a 1.5-fold increase in emergency LSCS rate when labour is induced or augmented.[3] Prostaglandins have the highest risk of uterine rupture (2.24%), although this may depend on the specific prostaglandin used; misoprostol carries the highest risk and therefore should be avoided as an induction agent in the third trimester.[2] Use of prostaglandins followed by oxytocin appears to increase the risk of rupture when compared with the single use of either agent.[2] The evidence for induction of labour after previous LSCS when the cervix is unfavourable is limited and conflicting, with some studies evaluated by ACOG indicating an increased risk of rupture or unsuccessful VBAC, while others have shown no significant difference.[2]

EXTERNAL CEPHALIC VERSION (ECV) AFTER PREVIOUS LSCS

By reducing the incidence of breech presentation at term, ECV lowers the overall rate of LSCS. Despite the theoretical risk of scar rupture during ECV in a woman who has had a previous LSCS, the chance of successful ECV is thought to be similar to that in women without a uterine scar.[2] ECV is therefore not an absolute contraindication,[3] although data are limited.

WHEN THERE IS DISAGREEMENT BETWEEN THE CLINICIAN AND WOMAN REGARDING MODE OF DELIVERY AFTER PREVIOUS CAESAREAN SECTION

There may be instances when a woman and her clinician significantly disagree about the recommended plan for delivery after a caesarean section. Examples could include a woman who is certain she wishes to go ahead with a trial of labour after three previous sections or when significant trauma such as a large extension occurred or a J-shaped incision was made at previous section. In these cases, the clinician should offer the woman a second opinion from a colleague either in the same unit or from a unit close by. The ultimate decision regarding the mode of delivery remains hers if she is deemed to have full mental capacity. Details of the discussions and counselling that have taken place should be fully documented in the medical notes, and the woman should be advised that the trial of labour should take place in a unit with facilities to manage potential catastrophic complications such as uterine rupture, with experienced surgeons and cell salvage.[2]

DELIVERY AFTER INTRAUTERINE FETAL DEATH IN THE SECOND TRIMESTER, OR TERMINATION OF PREGNANCY IN THE SECOND TRIMESTER, IN A WOMAN WITH A PREVIOUS LSCS

In the UK, misoprostol is the most commonly used agent to facilitate delivery after an intrauterine fetal death or for termination in the second trimester. However, when used in the third trimester it has been shown to significantly increase the risk of uterine rupture.[2] The data for the second-trimester deliveries was reassuring, however, and no significant difference in risk of rupture for women with or without a scarred uterus (less than 1%) was found.[2]

Reviewing local practice

As discussed, evidence on the safest mode of delivery for women with one or two LSCS is based largely on observational studies, rather than level 1 RCTs. It is important when counselling these women that local data are available when delivery options are discussed. Units should monitor their management of:

- caesarean sections in women with a previous LSCS: elective and emergency
- ECV rates: uptake and success
- VBAC rates: uptake, success, complications

These monitoring processes allow units to evaluate their services and care for women with a previous caesarean section, and help to identify areas where improvements need to be made, such as availability of VBAC workshops or training junior staff in counselling for mode of delivery.

Key summary points

- Endeavour to obtain as much information as possible about the previous caesarean section.
- Mode of delivery: VBAC and planned LSCS appear to be equally safe (from the evidence available) for a woman who has had a previous LSCS and has a singleton pregnancy with cephalic presentation and a straightforward antenatal course in her current pregnancy.
- It is important to take into account the woman's preference for mode of delivery, her attitude towards risk, and her motivation for a particular mode of delivery.
- Ensure the location of the placenta is identified in the antenatal period, and that if placenta praevia is present further investigations for accreta are arranged.
- The decision regarding mode of delivery should be clearly documented in the medical and handheld notes.

References

1. NHS Institute for Innovation and Improvement. Toolkit for reducing caesarean section rates. 2012. yhhiec.org.uk/wp-content/uploads/2012/01/1233_Toolkit_for_reducing_Caesarean_section_rates1.pdf (accessed 30 July 2015).

2. American College of Obstetricians and Gynecologists. Vaginal birth after previous cesarean delivery. *ACOG Practice Bulletin* August 2010; 115.

3. Royal College of Obstetricians and Gynaecologists. *Birth After Previous Caesarean Section*, 2nd edn. Green-top Guideline No. 45. London: RCOG, 2015.

4. National Institute for Health and Care Excellence (NICE). *Caesarean Section.* NICE Clinical Guideline CG132. London: NICE, 2011. www.nice.org.uk/guidance/cg132 (accessed 30 July 2015).

5. Dodd JM, Crowther CA, Huertas E, Guise JM, Horey D. Planned elective repeat caesarean section versus planned vaginal birth for women with a previous caesarean section birth. *Cochrane Database Syst Rev* 2013; (12): CD004224. DOI:10.1002/14651858.CD004224.pub2.

6. Glavind J, Kindberg SF, Uldberg N, *et al.* Elective caesarean section at 38 weeks versus 39 weeks: neonatal and maternal outcomes in a randomised controlled trial. *BJOG* 2013; 120: 1123–32.

Further reading

Grobman WA, Lai Y, Landon MB, *et al.* Can a prediction model for vaginal birth after caesarean section also predict the probability of morbidity related to trial of labor? *Am J Obstet Gynecol* 2009; 200(1): 56.el–56.e6. doi:10.1016/j.ajog.2008.06.039

Tita ATN, Landon MB, Spong CY, *et al.* Timing of elective repeat cesarean delivery at term and neonatal outcomes. *N Eng J Med.* 2009; 360: 111–20.

7 Common medical disorders in pregnancy

Shehnaaz Jivraj, Priya Madhuvrata, Sarah Vause, Remon Keriakos, and Frances Hills

7.1 ANAEMIA

Shehnaaz Jivraj

Background and clinical relevance

Iron-deficiency anaemia is the most common cause of anaemia worldwide. This review focuses on the management of iron-deficiency anaemia with a brief overview of the management of megaloblastic anaemias. It is compiled using standards set out by the National Institute for Health and Care Excellence (NICE) and the British Committee for Standards in Haematology (BCSH).

Only 15% of dietary iron is absorbed. Physiological iron requirements are three times higher in pregnancy than in menstruating women, increasing as pregnancy advances.[1]

Plasma volume increases by up to 15% by the end of the first trimester and by up to 50% by 34 weeks of pregnancy. There is a concomitant increase in red blood cell production which continues throughout pregnancy. However, a greater expansion of plasma volume relative to the increase in haemoglobin mass and erythrocyte volume is responsible for physiological or dilutional anaemia observed in healthy pregnant women.[2]

The fetal effects of anaemia range from intrauterine growth restriction, prematurity, infection and preterm rupture of membranes to intrauterine fetal death. Maternal consequences of anaemia include reduced physical and mental performance, reduced immunity, tiredness and an increased risk of postpartum haemorrhage and the need for blood transfusion.[3] It is for this reason that NICE recommends that all pregnant women should be offered screening for anaemia. This should take place early in pregnancy at the booking appointment, and at 28 weeks. This allows enough time for investigation and treatment if anaemia is

Antenatal Disorders for the MRCOG and Beyond, Second Edition, ed. Dilly Anumba and Shehnaaz Jivraj. Published by Cambridge University Press. © Cambridge University Press 2016.

detected. The normal UK lower limit for haemoglobin (Hb) in pregnancy is 11 g/dL in the first trimester and 10.5 g/dL at 28 weeks, and 10 g/dL in the postpartum period. Haemoglobin levels lower than this should be investigated, and iron supplementation considered if indicated. Iron supplements are not recommended routinely for all pregnant women, as they do not benefit the mother's or fetus's health and may have unpleasant maternal side effects such as gastric irritation and altered bowel habit.[4]

Treatment

ORAL IRON SUPPLEMENTS

When iron-deficiency anaemia is suspected on a full blood count, a trial of oral iron should be considered for 2 weeks, with an increment in haemoglobin demonstrated as a positive result. Thus a trial of oral iron can be used both as a diagnostic test and for treatment. Women with a known haemoglobinopathy should have serum ferritin checked, and they should be offered oral iron supplements if their ferritin level is < 30 µg/L. The recommended dose is 100–200 mg of elemental oral iron daily (Table 7.1.1). Appropriate advice on correct administration should be given to optimize absorption. Ideally, iron should be taken on an empty stomach, 1 hour before meals with a source of vitamin C. Antacids should be avoided. Foods rich in fibre and calcium slow absorption, as do coffee and caffeinated tea. In case of nausea or epigastric discomfort, lower doses of iron should be tried.

Once the haemoglobin is normalized, iron supplements should be taken for 3 months antenatally and 6 weeks postpartum.

Non-anaemic women (with a normal haemoglobin) who have a ferritin level of < 30 µg/L should also be offered oral iron supplements. Such women should be given 65 mg/day of elemental iron, and serum ferritin and haemoglobin repeated after 8 weeks.

Anaemic women may require additional precautions for delivery, such as delivery in a hospital setting, intravenous access, active management of the third stage of labour, plans for managing postpartum haemorrhage and blood group and save.

Table 7.1.1 Oral iron preparations[7]

Iron salt	Dose per tablet	Elemental iron
Ferrous fumarate	200 mg	65 mg
Ferrous gluconate	300 mg	35 mg
Ferrous sulphate (dried)	200 mg	65 mg
Ferrous sulphate	300 mg	60 mg
Sodium feredetate (Sytron)	190 mg / 5 mL elixir	27.5 mg / 5 mL

Postpartum women with a haemoglobin < 10 g/dL should be given 100–200 mg of elemental iron for 3 months with a repeat full blood count (FBC) and ferritin at the end of therapy to ensure Hb and iron stores are replete.

The World Health Organization (WHO) recommends universal supplementation with 60 mg/day of elemental iron from booking.[5] While this recommendation may be applicable in resource-poor settings, routine supplementation for all women in pregnancy is not recommended because of adverse fetal effects demonstrated in some studies.[6]

PARENTERAL IRON

Intravenous iron offers a rapid repletion of iron stores and raises haemoglobin levels over a short period of time. Compared to a blood transfusion it has a shorter infusion time (30 minutes vs. 2–4 hours per blood bag), is more cost-effective and has a lower risk profile. Parenteral iron should be considered from the second trimester onwards and during the postpartum period for women with confirmed iron deficiency who fail to respond to or are intolerant of oral iron.[7]

The preparations available in the UK are shown in Table 7.1.2. The different preparations have not been compared to each other in pregnancy. Iron III carboxymaltose (Ferinject) has an advantage of single intravenous administration using a standard dose of 1000 mg. Anaphylactic reactions can occur extremely rarely – 6 out of 10,000,000 vials used. Facilities for resuscitation and management of anaphylaxis should be available at hand.

Contraindications include first trimester of pregnancy, liver disease, active bacteraemia, anaemia not attributable to iron deficiency or conditions of iron overload such as haemosiderosis or haemochromatosis. Occasionally, side effects such as metallic taste, nausea, vomiting, headache, hypotension, muscular pain, fever and flushing have been reported. Ferinject should not be administered concomitantly with oral iron preparations (oral iron therapy should not start earlier than 5 days after the parenteral iron). An FBC should be checked 2 weeks after the infusion (for antenatal patients) prior to considering a second dose or restarting oral iron supplements. For postnatal patients the interval should be 6 weeks (less if the patient is symptomatic).

Table 7.1.2 Parenteral iron preparations

Generic name	Proprietary name
Iron (III) hydroxide dextran complex	Cosmofer
Iron (III) hydroxide sucrose complex	Venofer
Iron (III) carboxymaltose	Ferinject
Iron (III) isomaltoside	Monofer

Table 7.1.3   Indications for measuring serum ferritin[7]
Anaemic women where estimation of iron stores is necessary
Known haemoglobinopathy
Prior to parenteral iron replacement
Non-anaemic women with high risk of iron depletion
Previous anaemia
Multiparity $\geq$ para 3
Consecutive pregnancy <1 year following delivery
Vegetarians
Teenage pregnancies
Recent history of bleeding
Non-anaemic women where estimation of iron stores is necessary
High risk of bleeding
Women for whom a blood transfusion is absolutely unacceptable, e.g. on religious grounds

SERUM FERRITIN

While the routine use of ferritin as a measure of anaemia is not cost-effective, indications exist for measuring serum ferritin to assess iron stores (Table 7.1.3). Women with low iron stores are likely to become anaemic more quickly and so should have treatment to replenish iron stores.

BLOOD TRANSFUSION

This should be reserved for those with risk of further bleeding, imminent cardio-vascular compromise or symptoms requiring immediate attention. This should be underpinned by local guidelines and clear patient information.

Megaloblastic anaemias

Most megaloblastic anaemias result from a lack of either vitamin B_{12} or folate. One cause of megaloblastic anaemia in the UK is *pernicious anaemia*, in which lack of gastric intrinsic factor resulting from an autoimmune gastritis causes malabsorption of vitamin B_{12}. Apart from dietary deficiency, all other causes of vitamin B_{12} deficiency are attributable to malabsorption.

Hydroxocobalamin is the choice of vitamin B_{12} for therapy. It is retained in the body longer than cyanocobalamin and thus for maintenance therapy can be given at intervals of up to 3 months. For vitamin B_{12} deficiency, one recommended regime is to give 1 mg hydroxocobalamin by intramuscular injection three times a week for 2 weeks, followed by 1 mg at 3-monthly intervals. The initial 2 weeks of therapy should replenish deficiency, and subsequent 3-monthly injections prevent deficiency.

In *folate-deficient megaloblastic anaemia* daily folic acid supplementation for 4 months (5 mg once daily) brings about haematological remission and replenishes body stores in most instances. Folic acid should not be used in undiagnosed megaloblastic anaemia unless vitamin B_{12} is administered concurrently, otherwise neuropathy may be precipitated.

For the prevention of neural tube defects, folic acid 400 μg once daily is recommended for all women until 12 weeks of pregnancy. High-risk groups – namely, sickle cell disease, malabsorptive states such as coeliac patients, diabetic women, obese women and those with a personal (including partner) or family history of neural tube defects – are recommended folic acid 5 mg once daily until 12 weeks of pregnancy. Sickle cell patients should continue this throughout pregnancy.[8]

Key summary points

- Anaemia is a global problem.
- A 2-week trial of oral iron when iron deficiency is suspected is both diagnostic and therapeutic.
- Women with low ferritin but normal haemoglobin should have their iron stores replenished.
- Consideration should be given to parenteral iron in women close to delivery, or if oral iron is not tolerated.
- Blood transfusion has a role and should be backed by local policies and informed consent.

References

1. Tapiero H, Gate L, Tew KD. Iron: deficiencies and requirements. *Biomed Pharmacother* 2001; 55: 324–32.

2. Paidas MJ, Hossain N. Hematologic changes in pregnancy. In Paidas MJ, Hossain N, Shamsi T, *et al.*, eds. *Hemostasis and Thrombosis in Obstetrics and Gynaecology*. Oxford: Wiley-Blackwell, 2011, pp. 1–11.

3. Shamsi T. Red cell disorders. In Paidas MJ, Hossain N, Shamsi T, *et al.*, eds. *Hemostasis and Thrombosis in Obstetrics and Gynaecology*. Oxford: Wiley-Blackwell, 2011, pp. 12–27.

4. National Institute for Health and Care Excellence (NICE); National Collaborating Centre for Women's and Children's Health. *Antenatal Care: Routine Care for the Healthy Pregnant Woman*. NICE Clinical Guideline CG62. London: NICE, 2008.

5. World Health Organization. *Iron Deficiency Anaemia: Assessment, Prevention, and Control. A Guide for Programme Managers*. Geneva: WHO, 2001. http://www.who.int/nutrition/publications/en/ida_assessment_prevention_control.pdf (accessed 8 October 2015).

6. Ziaei S, Norrozi M, Faghihzadeh S, Jafarbegloo E. A randomised placebo-controlled trial to determine the effect of iron supplementation on pregnancy outcome in pregnant women with haemoglobin $\geq$ 13.2 g/dl. *BJOG* 2007; 114: 684–8.

7. Pavord S, Myers B, Robinson S, *et al.* UK guidelines on the management of iron deficiency in pregnancy. *Br J Haematol* 2012; 156: 588–600.

8. Joint Formulary Committee. *British National Formulary*, 66th ed. London: BMJ Group and Pharmaceutical Press, 2013.

7.2 ENDOCRINE DISORDERS

Priya Madhuvrata

Diabetes

BACKGROUND

Diabetes is a disorder of carbohydrate metabolism that requires immediate changes in lifestyle. Approximately 2–5% of pregnancies per year in England and Wales involve women with diabetes.[1] Pre-existing type 1 and type 2 diabetes account for 0.27% and 0.10% of births, respectively. The average prevalence of gestational diabetes mellitus (GDM) in England and Wales is approximately 3.5%. Insulin-dependent diabetes mellitus (IDDM, type 1) tends to present in children or young adults who are of normal weight. In contrast, non-insulin-dependent diabetes (NIDDM, type 2) occurs in an older and often overweight population.

EFFECT OF PREGNANCY ON DIABETES

Women with IDDM require increased doses of insulin during pregnancy, as pregnancy is a state of relative insulin resistance. Hormones secreted largely by the placenta, which include human placental lactogen, glucagon and cortisol, antagonize the effects of insulin. Often, by term, insulin requirements are two-fold greater than pre-pregnancy. As a result of tighter glucose control, episodes of hypoglycaemia are more common during pregnancy. Most women with nephropathy will experience no deterioration in renal function during pregnancy, although pregnancy may accelerate progression to end-stage kidney disease in some women with moderate to advanced diabetic nephropathy. Pregnancy appears to cause a worsening of diabetic retinopathy, which is more likely in women with more severe retinopathy, poor glycaemic control and hypertension.

EFFECT OF DIABETES ON PREGNANCY

Diabetes in pregnancy is associated with an increased incidence of complications (Table 7.2.1). There is an increased risk of congenital abnormality, two- to five-fold greater than in non-diabetic pregnancies, particularly cardiac, renal and neural tube defects. Sacral agenesis, which is specific to diabetic pregnancies, is rare. This increased risk of abnormality is related to maternal hyperglycaemia during embryogenesis and may be correlated with glycosylated haemoglobin. This emphasizes the importance of pre-pregnancy care to obtain optimal glycaemic control prior to conception. Miscarriage is more common in poorly controlled diabetics. Macrosomia is associated with poorly controlled disease but can occur in pregnancies with good glycaemic control, and intrauterine growth restriction is associated with women with microvascular disease.

Table 7.2.1 Adverse effects of diabetes on pregnancy

Congenital abnormality

Miscarriage

Pre-eclampsia

Preterm labour

Unexplained intrauterine death

Intrauterine growth restriction

Fetal macrosomia
- shoulder dystocia
- polyhydramnios
- increased caesarean section rate
- increased risk of metabolic disturbance in the fetus

Increased perinatal and neonatal mortality rates

Infection – urinary tract infection, vaginal candidiasis

Diabetic pregnancies are associated with increased perinatal and neonatal mortality rates about five times that in the general maternity population. With improvements in management and advances in neonatal care, the perinatal mortality in pregnancy complicated by diabetes has been reduced. However, the risk of unexplained intrauterine death, particularly in the late third trimester, remains.

MANAGEMENT OF DIABETIC PREGNANCY

Pre-pregnancy care

Pregnancy should be planned, and good contraceptive advice and pre-pregnancy counselling by a multidisciplinary team are essential. Good glycaemic control before conception and continuing this throughout pregnancy will reduce the risk of miscarriage, congenital malformation, stillbirth and neonatal death. The target for pre-pregnancy glycaemic control for most women should be an HbA1c < 7% (53 mmol/mol), although lower targets of HbA1c may be appropriate, as this is likely to reduce congenital malformations.[1]

Folic acid (5 mg/day) should be taken in the pre-conception period until 12 weeks of gestation to reduce the risk of having a baby with a neural tube defect. Women should be offered a meter for self-monitoring of blood glucose, to include fasting and a mixture of pre- and postprandial levels.[1]

Metformin and glibenclamide could be used in the pre-conception period and during pregnancy. All other oral hypoglycaemic agents should be discontinued before pregnancy and insulin substituted. Statins, angiotensin-converting enzyme (ACE) inhibitors and angiotensin receptor blocking medications should be discontinued before conception or as soon as pregnancy is confirmed. Retinal assessment and renal assessment should be offered before discontinuing contraception.[1,2]

Antenatal management

Antenatal care should be provided by a multidisciplinary team, led by a named obstetrician and physician with an interest in diabetes, and including a diabetes specialist nurse, diabetes specialist midwife and dietician.

Insulin therapy will require to be adjusted, usually switching from twice daily insulin to basal bolus regime. This usually takes the form of short-acting insulin preprandially before breakfast, lunch and dinner with intermediate or long-acting insulin in the morning and at night-time. Women should aim to keep fasting blood glucose between 3.5 and 5.9 mmol/L and 1-hour postprandial blood glucose below 7.8 mmol/L during pregnancy.[1] Women should be advised to test for ketonuria or ketonaemia if they become hyperglycaemic or unwell, to rule out diabetic ketoacidosis.

Hypoglycaemia is a relatively common occurrence, especially when tight diabetic control is the aim, and it is important that both the woman and her partner are aware of this risk and how to remedy the situation, using intramuscular glucagon injections when she is unable to eat. A low glycaemic index (GI) diet, exercise and calorie restriction in obese women improve glycaemic control.

Retinal assessment should be offered following the first antenatal clinic appointment and again at 28 weeks if the first assessment is normal. If any diabetic retinopathy is present, an additional retinal assessment should be performed at 16–20 weeks. Renal assessment should be arranged at the first contact in pregnancy. If serum creatinine is abnormal ($\geq$ 120 μmol/L) or if total protein excretion exceeds 2 g/day, referral to a nephrologist should be considered.[1] Women with diabetes should have contact with the diabetes care team for assessment of glycaemic control every 1–2 weeks throughout pregnancy. All women should be offered:

- an early viability scan
- a dating scan between 11 weeks and 13 weeks 6 days in association with biochemical screening and nuchal translucency measurement, to risk-assess for trisomies
- a detailed anomaly scan including four-chamber cardiac view and outflow tracts between 18 and 20 weeks
- ultrasound monitoring of fetal growth and amniotic fluid volume every 4 weeks from 28 to 36 weeks, to detect macrosomia, polyhydramnios or intrauterine growth restriction

Diabetes should not be considered a contraindication to antenatal steroids for fetal lung maturation, and to tocolysis. Women with insulin-treated diabetes who are receiving steroids for fetal lung maturation should have additional insulin according to an agreed protocol. Pregnant women with diabetes who have a normally grown fetus should be offered elective birth through induction of labour, or by elective caesarean section if indicated, after 38 completed weeks.

Intrapartum management

Intravenous dextrose and insulin infusion is recommended during labour and birth for women with diabetes whose blood glucose is not maintained at between 4 and 7 mmol/L. Both elective and emergency caesarean section rates are higher in these women, and this is partly explained by the associated higher median birth weight for gestation. The main hazard of vaginal delivery in women with diabetes is of shoulder dystocia with a macrosomic fetus. The risks of shoulder dystocia and brachial plexus injury are greater in infants of diabetic mothers than in similarly sized infants of non-diabetic mothers.

Following delivery of the placenta, the intravenous insulin infusion should be discontinued, and the pre-pregnancy insulin regimen recommenced. Women with pre-existing type 2 diabetes who are breastfeeding can resume or continue to take metformin and glibenclamide immediately after the birth.

The neonate will be at excess risk of problems such as hypoglycaemia, respiratory distress syndrome, polycythaemia and neonatal jaundice. Early breastfeeding is recommended to prevent neonatal hypoglycaemia.

GESTATIONAL DIABETES

Gestational diabetes can be defined as carbohydrate intolerance of variable severity with onset or first recognition during pregnancy. This definition will include women with abnormal glucose tolerance that reverts to normal after delivery, and those with undiagnosed type 1 or type 2 diabetes. Two randomized controlled trials (RCTs) have shown that intervention in women with gestational diabetes with dietary advice, monitoring and management of blood glucose is effective in reducing birth weight and the rate of large-for-gestational-age infants, as well as perinatal morbidity.[3,4] The most appropriate strategies for screening and diagnosing GDM remain controversial.

Screening at first antenatal visit

At booking, all women should be assessed for the presence of risk factors for gestational diabetes (Table 7.2.2).

All women with risk factors should have HbA1c or fasting glucose measured.

- Women in early pregnancy with levels of HbA1c $\geq$ 6.5% (48 mmol/mol), fasting glucose $\geq$ 7.0 mmol/L or 2-hour glucose $\geq$ 11.1 mmol/L, diagnostic of diabetes, should be treated as having pre-existing diabetes.
- Women with intermediate levels of glucose (HbA1c 6.0–6.4% or 42–46 mmol/mol), fasting glucose 5.1–6.9 mmol/L or 2-hour glucose 8.5–11.0 mmol/L should be assessed to determine the need for immediate home glucose monitoring and, if the diagnosis remains unclear, assessed for gestational diabetes by 75 g oral glucose tolerance test (OGTT) at 24–28 weeks.[2,5]

Table 7.2.2   Risk factors for gestational diabetes: women with any one of these risk factors should be offered testing for gestational diabetes

Body mass index (BMI) > 30 kg/m^2

Previous macrosomic baby weighing ≥ 4.5 kg

Previous gestational diabetes

Family history of diabetes (first-degree relative with diabetes)

Family origin with a high prevalence of diabetes:
- South Asian (specifically women whose country of family origin is India, Pakistan or Bangladesh)
- Black Caribbean
- Middle Eastern (specifically women whose country of family origin is Saudi Arabia, United Arab Emirates, Iraq, Jordan, Syria, Oman, Qatar, Kuwait, Lebanon or Egypt)

Screening later in pregnancy

All women with risk factors should have a 75 g OGTT at 24–28 weeks.

Diagnosis of gestational diabetes

The International Association of Diabetes in Pregnancy recommends 75 g OGTT, with gestational diabetes diagnosed where one or more threshold value is exceeded (fasting venous plasma glucose ≥ 5.1 mmol/L, 1-hour value ≥ 10 mmol/L, 2-hour ≥ 8.5 mmol/L).[5] NICE and WHO diagnostic levels are fasting plasma glucose ≥ 5.6 mmol/L, or at 2 hours ≥ 7.8 mmol/L following 75 g OGTT.[1]

Importance of gestational diabetes

- Increased risk of having a baby who is large for gestational age, which increases the likelihood of birth trauma, induction of labour and caesarean section.
- The possibility of transient morbidity in the baby during the neonatal period, which may require admission to the neonatal unit.
- The risk of the baby developing obesity and/or diabetes in later life.

Women identified as having gestational diabetes should attend specialist clinics managed by both obstetricians and physicians. Lifestyle advice including dietary modification is the primary intervention. If diet and exercise fail to maintain blood glucose targets during a period of 1–2 weeks, oral hypoglycaemic agents (metformin or glibenclamide) should be considered as an initial hypoglycaemic agent.[1,2] Supplemental insulin may be required, depending on glycaemic control.

Women with gestational diabetes are at increased risk of pre-eclampsia, and their blood pressure and urinalysis should be checked regularly. Ultrasound monitoring of fetal growth and amniotic fluid volume should be carried out every 4 weeks from 28 to 36 weeks to detect macrosomia and polyhydramnios, which may influence the mode of delivery if macrosomia is identified. Women requiring insulin or oral glucose-lowering medication who have pregnancies which are otherwise progressing normally should be assessed at 38 weeks gestation with delivery shortly after, and certainly by 40 weeks.[2] Early feeding is advised to avoid neonatal hypoglycaemia. All hypoglycaemic agents should be stopped following delivery.

Women should be informed about the risks of gestational diabetes in future pregnancies and type 2 diabetes in later life. They should be offered lifestyle advice (including weight control, diet and exercise) and offered a fasting plasma glucose measurement at the 6-week postnatal check and annually thereafter.[1]

KEY SUMMARY POINTS

- A multidisciplinary team, led by a named obstetrician and physician with an interest in diabetes, and including a diabetes specialist nurse, diabetes specialist midwife and dietician, should provide care from pre-pregnancy to postnatal review.
- Good glycaemic control before conception and continuing this throughout pregnancy will reduce the risk of miscarriage, congenital malformation, stillbirth and neonatal death.
- The target for pre-pregnancy glycaemic control for most women should be an HbA1c of less than 7% (53 mmol/mol).
- Folic acid (5 mg/day) should be taken in the pre-conception period until 12 weeks of gestation.
- Insulin therapy during pregnancy will require to be adjusted, usually switching from twice-daily insulin to basal bolus regime (background and pre-meal insulin). Metformin and glibenclamide could be used in the pre-conception period and during pregnancy.
- Pregnant women with diabetes who have a normally grown fetus should be offered elective birth through induction of labour after 38 completed weeks. The main hazard of vaginal delivery is shoulder dystocia with a macrosomic fetus.
- Women with gestational diabetes should be offered lifestyle advice (including weight control, diet and exercise) and offered a fasting plasma glucose measurement at the 6-week postnatal check and annually thereafter due to increased risk of type 2 diabetes in future.

Thyroid disease

PHYSIOLOGY

During pregnancy, increased circulating oestrogen levels stimulate the hepatic production of thyroid-binding globulin (TBG). To compensate for this rise in TBG, total levels of circulating tri-iodothyronine (T_3) and thyroxine (T_4) are increased. An evaluation of thyroid function during pregnancy therefore requires an assessment of free T_3 and free T_4. Both free T_3 and free T_4 are slightly elevated in the first trimester, and thyroid-stimulating hormone (TSH) is decreased; in 10–15% of normal women, TSH is suppressed into the hyperthyroid range. This may, in part, be due to placental production of human chorionic gonadotrophin (hCG), which is structurally similar to TSH and does have some thyrotrophic activity. In the third trimester of pregnancy, concentrations of free T_3 and free T_4 are reduced, and TSH concentration is increased.

HYPERTHYROIDISM

Hyperthyroidism is a relatively common medical condition, which occurs in around 1 in 500 pregnancies. Most (95%) are secondary to Graves' disease, an autoimmune disorder where the thyroid is stimulated by antibodies directed against the TSH receptor. The diagnosis of hyperthyroidism is made biochemically, by detecting a raised free T_3 or free T_4. TSH levels will be suppressed, although this can occur in normal pregnancy.

Effect of pregnancy on hyperthyroidism
Like most autoimmune conditions, Graves' disease often improves during pregnancy, although the increased thyroid activity that occurs in the first trimester can worsen the disease. An exacerbation can also occur postpartum, and this is associated with increasing levels of TSH receptor-stimulating antibodies (TRAb).

Effect of hyperthyroidism on pregnancy
Well-controlled patients rarely have problems during pregnancy. Those with uncontrolled disease have an increased risk of spontaneous miscarriage, intrauterine growth restriction, preterm delivery and increased perinatal mortality. Other fetal problems relate to the transfer of TRAb from mother to fetus, which can provoke fetal hyperthyroidism (0.01%) and neonatal thyrotoxicosis (10%). The major risk to the mother is congestive cardiac failure and a thyroid crisis. These complications can be precipitated by infection or stress and are characterized by tachycardia and hyperpyrexia, vomiting, diarrhoea and central nervous system dysfunction. Rarely, a goitre can enlarge during pregnancy to cause a degree of tracheal obstruction that may be detected only during intubation.

Management of hyperthyroidism
Carbimazole and propylthiouracil are the antithyroid drugs most commonly used in the UK, and methimazole, a metabolite of carbimazole, is the drug most commonly employed in the USA. The dose of antithyroid drugs should be adjusted to maintain the maternal free T_4 at or just above the upper limit of the reference range.[6] Both drugs readily cross the placenta, and, although neither is teratogenic, carbimazole has been associated with a rare scalp defect, aplasia cutis. Carbimazole and propylthiouracil will affect the fetal thyroid, and, in high doses, these drugs may cause fetal hypothyroidism and goitre. Maternal adverse effects include skin rash (1%), arthralgia and gastrointestinal symptoms. The most serious adverse

effect is granulocytopenia, usually dose-related and occurring within 2 months of commencing treatment. Women should be advised to report a skin rash or sore throat immediately. Propylthiouracil may be associated with severe liver toxicity, and therefore it is reasonable to monitor liver function every 4 weeks.

TRAb freely cross the placenta and can stimulate the fetal thyroid. These antibodies should be measured by 22 weeks gestational age in mothers with current Graves' disease, a history of Graves' disease, or treatment with iodine-131 or thyroidectomy before pregnancy. In women with elevated TRAb, fetal thyroid dysfunction (thyroid enlargement, growth restriction, hydrops) should be screened for during the fetal anatomy ultrasound.

Antithyroid drugs can be continued during breastfeeding. Since less pro-pylthiouracil crosses the placenta and is excreted in breastmilk, this drug is preferable for hyperthyroidism in pregnancy. Carbimazole and methimazole are excreted in breastmilk in significant amounts but do not seem to alter neonatal thyroid function in low doses ($<$ 30 mg/day).

Beta-blockers are commonly employed to control tachycardia and tremor. These agents should be discontinued, since long-term administration is associated with intrauterine growth restriction. Surgery is indicated where patients do not respond to drug therapy, in cases of thyroid carcinoma, or where an enlarging goitre is compressing surrounding structures. The optimal timing of surgery is in the second trimester. Radioactive iodine therapy is contraindicated during pregnancy and for mothers who are breastfeeding, since the radioiodine is sequestered by the fetal thyroid gland, resulting in ablation and hypothyroidism. Pregnancy should not be contemplated for at least 4 months after radioiodine treatment.

HYPOTHYROIDISM

Hypothyroidism occurs in 0.3–0.5% of pregnancies. Chronic autoimmune thyroiditis is the main cause of hypothyroidism, apart from iodine deficiency, radio-iodine ablation or thyroidectomy, and congenital hypothyroidism. The diagnosis is confirmed biochemically by identifying a low free T_4 and a raised TSH. In the first trimester, the 'normal' range of TSH is reduced to 0.1–2.5 mIU/L. Trimester-specific reference ranges should be used for pregnant women if using a free T_4 assay.

Levothyroxine is the treatment of choice for maternal hypothyroidism. Thyroid function should be monitored at least once per trimester to ensure adequate replacement of thyroxine.

Effect of pregnancy on hypothyroidism
Pregnancy has little or no effect on hypothyroidism.

Effect of hypothyroidism on pregnancy
It is unusual for hypothyroidism to cause significant problems in pregnancy. Severe and untreated disease is associated with an increased risk of spontaneous

miscarriage, perinatal mortality, pre-eclampsia, premature birth and intrauterine growth restriction. Thyroid hormone contributes critically to normal fetal brain development. Children born to untreated hypothyroid mothers were three times more likely to have IQs that were 1 SD below the mean of controls.[6]

Management of hypothyroidism

Women receiving thyroxine prior to pregnancy usually should increase their dosage by 4–6 weeks gestation to 30–50% above pre-conception dosage. Thyroid function tests are then monitored at least in each trimester, with dose adjustment if TSH is elevated and free T_4 low. If overt hypothyroidism is diagnosed during pregnancy, thyroid function tests should be normalized as rapidly as possible. Thyroxine dosage should be titrated to rapidly reach and thereafter maintain serum TSH concentrations of less than 2.5 mIU/L.[6] Thyroid function should be re-measured within 4–6 weeks. After delivery, most hypothyroid women need to decrease the thyroxine dosage to their pre-pregnancy dose.

KEY SUMMARY POINTS

- Trimester-specific reference ranges should be used for pregnant women if using a free T_3 and T_4 assay.
- Less propylthiouracil crosses the placenta and is excreted in breastmilk, so this drug is preferable for hyperthyroidism in pregnancy.
- Levothyroxine is the treatment of choice for maternal hypothyroidism. Thyroid function tests should be monitored at least once per trimester to ensure adequate replacement of thyroxine.

Prolactinoma

Pregnancy is normally associated with a substantial increase in circulating prolactin levels of around 10–20-fold. There is also an increase in volume of the pituitary gland (up to 35%) during pregnancy. These elevated levels of prolactin return to normal when breastfeeding is discontinued.

EFFECT OF PREGNANCY ON PROLACTINOMA

Prolactinomas are the most commonly encountered pituitary tumours in pregnancy. They can be either microprolactinomas (< 1 cm) or macroprolactinomas (> 1 cm). Since the pituitary gland enlarges during pregnancy, there is a small risk that the oestrogenic stimulation will provoke tumour expansion, leading to headache, visual field defects or the development of diabetes insipidus. It is unusual for patients with microadenomas to have a clinically significant expansion in their tumour during pregnancy (risk $< 2\%$), although the risk for macroadenomas is much greater (15%). This latter figure can be reduced (to $< 5\%$) if the tumour has been treated prior to conception.

EFFECT OF PROLACTINOMA ON PREGNANCY

Women with hyperprolactinaemia due to prolactinoma will clearly have a problem with fertility, although ovulation is likely to return to normal following treatment with the dopamine receptor agonists bromocriptine or cabergoline.

MANAGEMENT OF PROLACTINOMA

Dopamine agonist therapy should be discontinued when these patients become pregnant. In selected patients with macroadenomas who become pregnant on dopaminergic therapy and who have not had prior surgical or radiation therapy, it may be prudent to continue dopaminergic therapy throughout the pregnancy. The patient should be made aware of the risk of tumour expansion and the need to report severe headache or change in vision during the pregnancy.[7]

Monitoring of prolactin levels during pregnancy is not recommended. For most pregnant patients with prolactinomas, serial MRIs and formal visual field testing are not indicated in the absence of headaches or visual field changes. For patients who have macroadenomas and have not undergone prior pituitary surgery, it is prudent to undertake more frequent clinical examinations and formal visual field testing.[7] Should symptoms occur, tumour size and expansion should be determined by magnetic resonance imaging; dopamine receptor agonists can be reintroduced with no adverse effects on the pregnancy. Breastfeeding is not contraindicated in patients with prolactinomas or in women on dopamine receptor agonists, although these agents may inhibit milk production.

KEY SUMMARY POINTS

- Dopamine agonist therapy should be discontinued when patients with prolactinoma become pregnant.
- There is risk of expansion of prolactinoma during pregnancy, and the patient should be advised to report severe headache or change in vision.

References

1. National Institute for Health and Care Excellence (NICE). *Diabetes in Pregnancy: Management from Preconception to the Postnatal Period.* NICE Guideline NG3. London: NICE, 2015.

2. Scottish Intercollegiate Guidelines Network (SIGN). *Management of Diabetes: a National Clinical Guideline.* SIGN Guideline No. 116. Edinburgh: SIGN, 2010.

3. Crowther CA, Hiller JE, Moss JR, *et al.*; Australian Carbohydrate Intolerance Study in Pregnant Women (ACHOIS) Trial Group. Effect of treatment of gestational diabetes mellitus on pregnancy outcomes. *N Engl J Med* 2005; 352: 2477–86.

4. Landon MB, Spong CY, Thom E, *et al.* A multicenter, randomized trial of treatment for mild gestational diabetes. *N Engl J Med* 2009; 361: 1339–48.

5. International Association of Diabetes and Pregnancy Study Groups Consensus Panel. International association of diabetes and pregnancy study groups recommendations on the diagnosis and classification of hyperglycemia in pregnancy. *Diabetes Care* 2010; 33: 676–82.

6. De Groot L, Abalovich M, Alexander EK, *et al.* Management of thyroid dysfunction during pregnancy and postpartum: an Endocrine Society clinical practice guideline. *J Clin Endocrinol Metab* 2012; 97: 2543–65.

7. Melmed S, Casanueva FF, Hoffman AR, *et al.* Diagnosis and treatment of hyperprolactinemia: an Endocrine Society clinical practice guideline. *J Clin Endocrinol Metab* 2011; 96: 273–88.

Further reading

HAPO Study Cooperative Research Group. Hyperglycemia and adverse pregnancy outcomes. *N Engl J Med* 2008; 358: 1991–2002.

7.3 GASTROINTESTINAL AND HEPATIC DISEASE

Priya Madhuvrata

Physiological changes during pregnancy

Gastrointestinal motility is reduced during pregnancy, with delayed gastric emptying and reduced bowel transit times. There is a reduction in distal oesophageal pressure. These changes mean that heartburn, nausea, vomiting and constipation are common during normal pregnancy. There is an increase in liver metabolism during pregnancy. Alkaline phosphatase rises during pregnancy, mainly due to increased production by the placenta, but the other liver enzymes are largely unchanged. For the transaminases, γ-glutamyl transferase and bilirubin, the upper limit of normal throughout pregnancy is 20% lower than the non-pregnant range.

Reflux oesophagitis

Oesophagitis arises from reflux of gastric contents into the lower oesophagus, which results in inflammation. This is extremely common, because of the reduction in lower oesophageal pressure and delayed gastric emptying during pregnancy. The enlarging gravid uterus exacerbates the condition in late pregnancy. Reflux most commonly presents with heartburn, nausea and vomiting. Less often, the woman with reflux will present with haematemesis or respiratory symptoms. Postural changes, particularly at night with elevation of the head of the bed, and dietary modifications may be helpful. The pharmacological management of reflux includes antacid preparations, sucralfate, and the histamine receptor antagonists (H$_2$RAs) ranitidine and metoclopramide. Proton pump inhibitors should only be used during pregnancy in women who do not respond to lifestyle changes, antacids and H_2RAs.

Peptic ulcer disease

Peptic ulcer disease is traditionally thought to occur less commonly during pregnancy. This may be explained by a protective effect of pregnancy-induced prostaglandins on the gastric mucosa. Alternatively, the incidence of peptic ulcer disease during pregnancy may be underestimated because of a reluctance to perform endoscopy and an eagerness on the part of clinicians to ascribe symptoms to reflux. The presenting symptoms of peptic ulcer disease include epigastric pain, nausea and vomiting; gastrointestinal haemorrhage and perforation are extremely uncommon during pregnancy. The diagnosis is confirmed by endoscopy, which can be performed during pregnancy and is indicated when epigastric pain complicates nausea, vomiting and heartburn. The management includes antacids, sucralfate, ranitidine and proton pump inhibitors.[1] Both H_2RAs and proton pump inhibitors are safe and appropriate to use if required in pregnancy, as is conventional triple therapy for *Helicobacter pylori* eradication. Endoscopy during pregnancy is safe and is appropriate to perform if clinically indicated. When peptic ulcers have remained quiescent during pregnancy, a postpartum exacerbation in symptoms is not uncommon. It is important that epigastric pain in pregnancy is never attributed to a gastrointestinal problem until pre-eclampsia has been excluded.

Inflammatory bowel disease (Crohn's disease and ulcerative colitis)

This tends to present in young adulthood (20–40 years), and has an incidence of approximately 10 per 100,000. Crohn's disease can affect any part of the gastrointestinal tract but has a particular tendency to affect the terminal ileum, while ulcerative colitis is always confined to the colon. There is overlap between these two conditions in their clinical, histological and radiological features.

Most women with inflammatory bowel disease find that pregnancy has little effect on the course of their disease. The outcome is best if the disease is quiescent at the time of conception. Exacerbation of ulcerative colitis tends to occur in the first half of pregnancy, while increased disease activity in Crohn's most commonly presents in the first trimester. Exacerbation is more common in women who conceive during periods of active disease, and a postpartum flare may occur with Crohn's disease.

For the majority of women, the disease has no effect on their pregnancy. Active disease early in pregnancy is associated with spontaneous miscarriage and, later in pregnancy, with an increased risk of preterm delivery. Women who have previously undergone surgical management cope well with pregnancy and labour, although transient ileostomy dysfunction may occur from mid-pregnancy. This often resolves with fasting and intravenous fluids. Acute inflammatory bowel disease is an important risk factor for venous thromboembolism.

Pre-pregnancy counselling is important, since women should be encouraged to postpone conception until their disease is quiescent. Mycophenolate and methotrexate should be stopped and replaced with a suitable alternative at least 3 months before conception. For women who have recently used methotrexate or sulphasalazine (SASP), high-dose folate supplementation, 5 mg once daily, is recommended.[2]

Disease activity during pregnancy can be managed with SASP and corticosteroids given orally and by enema. Azathioprine (AZA) can be safely used in pregnancy. With the exception of mycophenolate and methotrexate, medication should continue, with indications unchanged from the non-pregnant state, as the risks associated with active disease outweigh those of continued treatment. There are insufficient data to recommend the use of biologics such as infliximab in pregnancy, and in practice this can be unavoidable for patients with severe refractory disease.[2] Most women becoming pregnant while on biologics have probably gained a remission using such agents and the risk–benefit balance almost certainly falls strongly in favour of continuing treatment. When complications of the disease arise (perforation, obstruction, abscess formation, toxic megacolon), surgery may be required.

Delivery by caesarean section should be reserved for obstetric indications, for women with perianal Crohn's, and for cases where an ileoanal anastomosis and pouch is in place. Thrombotic risk should be considered and thromboprophylaxis instituted where multiple risk factors are present. The literature shows no evidence of harm with SASP, AZA and infliximab, although the drug manufacturers generally suggest avoiding breastfeeding.

Intrahepatic cholestasis of pregnancy

Intrahepatic cholestasis of pregnancy (ICP, also known as obstetric cholestasis) is associated with an increased incidence of adverse maternal and fetal outcomes. The prevalence of the condition in the UK is 0.5–1%, although it may be as high as 12% in certain populations, such as in Chile, South America. The pathogenesis of ICP is incompletely understood, although there appears to be a genetic predisposition to the cholestatic effect of elevated circulating oestrogen.

ICP is diagnosed when otherwise unexplained pruritus occurs in pregnancy and abnormal liver function tests (LFTs) and/or raised bile acids occur in the pregnant woman and both resolve after delivery. Pruritus that involves the palms and soles of the feet is particularly suggestive. In those with persistent unexplained pruritus and normal biochemistry, LFTs should be measured every 1–2 weeks. Other causes of pruritus and abnormal LFTs should be sought. This may include carrying out a viral screen for hepatitis A, B and C, Epstein–Barr and cytomegalovirus, a liver autoimmune screen for chronic active hepatitis and primary biliary cirrhosis (anti-smooth muscle and anti-mitochondrial antibodies) and liver ultrasound.

Fetal risks associated with ICP include spontaneous preterm labour, intracranial haemorrhage, meconium staining, intrauterine fetal death and intrapartum fetal distress. Older series have reported a stillbirth rate of about 10%, although more recent series, where women were electively delivered by 38 weeks of gestation, indicate that this rate has reduced to 1–2%.[3] However, there has been little change in the reported rates of preterm labour (30–40%) and meconium staining (25–35%). The maternal risks of ICP include vitamin K deficiency (with subsequent disturbed coagulation) and an increased risk of antepartum haemorrhage. Further, these women have a significant risk (35%) of pruritus on combined oral contraceptives.

The management of ICP is to establish the diagnosis by excluding other causes of cholestasis (including viral hepatitis, gallstones and primary biliary cirrhosis) and then to counsel the mother about the adverse sequelae that are associated with the condition. Liver function tests, bile acids and a coagulation screen should be assessed weekly. Antihistamines may relieve pruritus. Ursodeoxycholic acid (UDCA) improves pruritus and liver function in women with ICP, but there is lack of robust data concerning protection against stillbirth and safety to the fetus or neonate.[3] Dexamethasone should not be first-line therapy for treatment of ICP, nor should it be used outside of a randomized controlled trial (RCT). If the prothrombin time is prolonged, the use of water-soluble vitamin K (menadiol sodium phosphate) in doses of 5–10 mg daily is indicated. When prothrombin time is normal, vitamin K in low doses should be used only after careful counselling about the likely benefits (less risk of maternal and fetal haemorrhage) but small theoretical risk (risk of neonatal haemolytic anaemia, hyperbilirubinaemia and kernicterus). While the benefits of fetal surveillance are uncertain, most units perform cardiotocography and ultrasound scans for amniotic fluid volume, fetal growth and biophysical profile scores, and Doppler studies. Early delivery, usually by induction of labour, should be undertaken after 37 weeks of gestation, because of inability to predict stillbirth if pregnancy continues.

LFTs should be checked 6 weeks after delivery to ensure that they are normal, with a postnatal review for reassurance about the lack of long-term sequelae for mother and baby, and for discussions of the high recurrence rate (45–90%), contraceptive choices (usually avoiding oestrogen-containing methods) and the increased incidence of ICP in family members.

Acute fatty liver of pregnancy

Acute fatty liver of pregnancy (AFLP) is a rare condition with an approximate incidence of 1 in 7,000 to 1 in 20,000 pregnancies; it may be a variant of pre-eclampsia. A comprehensive review by the UK Obstetric Surveillance System (UKOSS) found 57 cases in 1,132,964 maternities.[4] It is a serious condition with high maternal and fetal mortality: 15% and 25%, respectively. Earlier studies reported maternal mortality rates of 80–90%. The condition is associated with an inherited deficiency of a mitochondrial enzyme, long-chain 3-hydroxyacetyl coenzyme-A dehydrogenase (LCHAD). This enzyme catalyses a reaction in the β-oxidation of fatty acids, and so deficiency allows the build-up of long-chain fatty acids. LCHAD deficiency is an autosomal recessive disorder, and often the mother will be heterozygous for the abnormal gene with a homozygous fetus producing the excessive toxic metabolites. However, not all women who carry fetuses with the abnormal genotype will go on to develop liver disease. It is thought that other stressors, such as pre-eclampsia, increase the risk of developing AFLP.

The condition usually presents in the third trimester with symptoms of nausea, malaise and vomiting; abdominal pain may subsequently develop. The features of pre-eclampsia (proteinuria and hypertension) are often present, and the condition has to be differentiated from HELLP syndrome. Liver function tests are abnormal, with raised transaminases, alkaline phosphatase and bilirubin. In contrast to HELLP syndrome, AFLP is associated with a marked hypoglycaemia, leucocytosis and hyperuricaemia. Fulminant hepatic failure with encephalopathy, disseminated intravascular coagulation and renal failure may develop.

Liver histology shows microvesicular fatty infiltration of hepatocytes, especially in the central zone. However, liver biopsy is often omitted since it can be hazardous, especially in the presence of coagulopathy. The management goal for AFLP is correction of any coagulopathy and hypoglycaemia and prompt delivery. These women may deteriorate rapidly, and their management should involve a multidisciplinary team. Plasmapheresis is recommended in some reports, and N-acetylcysteine (a glutathione precursor and antioxidant) may be used to promote the selective inactivation of free radicals in hepatic failure. In the most severe cases involving fulminant hepatic failure and encephalopathy, the patient should be urgently transferred to a specialist liver unit and liver transplantation considered.

Key summary points

- In women with inflammatory bowel disease, mycophenolate and methotrexate should be stopped and replaced with suitable alternatives at least 3 months before conception. Azathioprine can be safely used in pregnancy.
- Intrahepatic cholestasis of pregnancy (ICP, obstetric cholestasis) is diagnosed when otherwise unexplained pruritus occurs in pregnancy, abnormal liver function tests and/or raised bile acids occur, and all clinical features resolve after delivery.
- Induction of labour should be undertaken in women with ICP after 37 weeks of gestation, as stillbirth cannot be predicted if pregnancy continues.
- Liver function tests are abnormal in acute fatty liver of pregnancy (AFLP), with raised transaminases, alkaline phosphatase and bilirubin. In contrast to HELLP syndrome, AFLP is associated with a marked hypoglycaemia, leucocytosis and hyperuricaemia.
- The management of AFLP entails correction of any coagulopathy and hypoglycaemia and prompt delivery.

References

1. Frise CJ, Nelson-Piercy C. Peptic ulcer disease in pregnancy. *J Obstet Gynaecol* 2012; 32: 804–11.

2. Crohn's and Colitis UK. *Pregnancy and IBD*, edition 6a. St Albans: Crohn's and Colitis UK, 2013.

3. Royal College of Obstetricians and Gynaecologists. *Obstetric Cholestasis*. Green-top Guideline No. 43. London: RCOG, 2011.

4. Knight M. Acute fatty liver of pregnancy in the UK: A national study to describe disease incidence, prognostic factors, management and outcomes. On behalf of UK Obstetric Surveillance System (UKOSS). 2007.

7.4 HAEMATOLOGICAL DISORDERS

Shehnaaz Jivraj

Introduction

This section is centred on problems commonly encountered in an obstetric haematology clinic and addresses problems that an obstetrician is likely to encounter in everyday clinical practice.

Haemoglobinopathies

The haemoglobin molecule is a tetramer consisting of four polypeptide chains known as globins. Normal adult haemoglobin, HbA, consists of two α chains and two β chains. Attached to each chain is an iron-containing molecule known as haem. Oxygen is transported in combination with the iron molecule of the haem group via a reversible oxygenation reaction. Lack of iron or abnormalities in the structure of the globin chains can result in impairment of oxygen carriage by the haemoglobin molecule.

Fetal haemoglobin, HbF ($\alpha_2\gamma_2$), represents 90–95% of all haemoglobin by 34–36 weeks gestation. Adult haemoglobin, HbA ($\alpha_2\beta_2$), accounts for 4–13% of total haemoglobin in the fetus. After 34 weeks gestation, HbA production increases significantly as HbF production falls. At term, HbF represents 53–95% of all haemoglobin, with HbA levels reaching 20–30%. In addition to being increased in some haemoglobinopathies, increased levels of HbF can be seen in infants who are small for gestational age, who have experienced chronic hypoxia, or who have trisomy 13.

Haemoglobin F percentage remains static for the first 2 weeks of life and then decreases by approximately 3% per week when erythropoiesis recommences, and is normally < 2–3% of total haemoglobin by 6 months of age. HbA becomes the predominant haemoglobin by 3 months of age, although this switch may be delayed in sick preterm infants.

Haemoglobin A_2 ($\alpha_2\delta_2$) is produced in small amounts from birth and usually reaches adult levels by 6 months of age, although it can rise further for the first 1–2 years of life. HbA_2 and Hb Bart's (γ_4 tetramers) may be detected in normal infants born at term.

The pattern of haemoglobin synthesis during development explains why α-chain abnormalities cause clinical problems from early fetal life, and why β-chain abnormalities may be difficult to diagnose in the neonatal period.[1]

Iron deficiency has been addressed in Section 7.1, above. In this section, we shall discuss sickle cell and thalassaemia – the most common haemoglobinopathies encountered in clinical practice.

Haemoglobinopathies are common in people whose family origins are in malarial parts of the world. In the UK, haemoglobinopathies are seen particularly among minority ethnic groups from Africa, the Caribbean, the Mediterranean, the Middle East, Southeast Asia and East Asia. Approximately 1000 haemoglobin variants have been identified worldwide.

Sickle cell disease

Sickle cell disease (SCD) is the name given to a group of inherited conditions of haemoglobin formation. SCD includes sickle cell anaemia (HbSS) and the heterozygous conditions of haemoglobin S and other clinically abnormal haemoglobins. These include combination with haemoglobin C, giving HbSC; combination with β-thalassaemia, giving HbSβ-thalassaemia; and combination with haemoglobin D, E or O-Arab. All these genotypes will give a similar clinical phenotype of varying severity. Haemoglobin S combined with haemoglobin A (HbAS), also known as sickle trait, is asymptomatic except for a possible increased risk of urinary tract infections.[2]

Under low oxygen conditions the abnormal haemoglobin polymerizes, leading to the formation of rigid and fragile sickle-shaped erythrocytes which are prone to increased breakdown, causing haemolytic anaemia; and to vaso-occlusion of small blood vessels, causing acute painful crises, end-organ damage and other complications.

Although the sickle gene is found in all ethnic groups, most people affected are of African or African-Caribbean origin. SCD can have a significant impact on morbidity and mortality. It is estimated that 240,000 people are carriers and between 12,500 and 15,000 people have SCD in the UK.[3] The prevalence of the disease is increasing because of immigration into the UK and new births. It is estimated to affect 1 in every 2000 births in England. Through the NHS Sickle Cell and Thalassaemia (SCT) Screening Programme, more cases are being diagnosed. Every year, approximately 360 newborn babies are identified with screen-positive results for significant condition, and over 9600 babies are identified as a carrier of a haemoglobin variant.

Because of progress in the management of the condition, children with SCD in the UK are now living to reproductive age, with an average life expectancy in the mid-fifties.[4]

Beta-thalassaemia

There are approximately 214,000 carriers in the UK, with 700 people affected by thalassaemia major (β-thalassaemia). Here the body is unable to produce normal haemoglobin, leading to life-threatening anaemia. Affected individuals require regular blood transfusions and chelation therapy to prevent complications of iron overload. The highest carrier prevalence is among Cypriot, Italian, Greek, Indian, Pakistani, Bangladeshi, Chinese, other Southeast Asian and Middle Eastern populations.

Both SCD and thalassaemia major can have effects on pregnancy and restrict a child's ability to function normally.

Antenatal screening

The antenatal screening policy in England is to offer sickle cell and thalassaemia screening to all women as part of early antenatal care. The purpose is to identify at-risk couples in order to offer an informed choice of prenatal diagnosis.

Two approaches are used, depending on whether the antenatal unit is in a high-prevalence (fetal prevalence of SCD $\geq$ 1.5 per 10,000 pregnancies) or low-prevalence (fetal prevalence of SCD $<$ 1.5 per 10,000 pregnancies) area.

In high-prevalence areas, a blood sample is sent to the laboratory for full blood count (FBC) and high-performance liquid chromatography (HPLC) or a suitable alternative technique such as haemoglobin electrophoresis on a maternal blood sample. A family-origin questionnaire (FOQ) is also completed and sent to the laboratory. It is recommended that testing of the women should ideally be completed before 12 weeks of pregnancy. In low-prevalence areas, the FOQ is used to determine the couple's family origin. An FBC is sent and the red cell indices are analysed and acted on as for high-prevalence areas. Haemoglobin analysis is confined to those women whose own origin, or whose baby's father's origin, is not northern European or is unknown.

Antenatal screening identifies about 22,000 carriers of SCD and thalassaemia every year.[5]

Management of sickle cell disease in pregnancy

PRE-CONCEPTION CARE

The consultation should be with a sickle specialist. The purpose of pre-conception care is to:

1. Inform the woman of how SCD can affect pregnancy and how pregnancy can affect SCD.

   SCD is associated with both maternal and fetal complications. Maternal complications include acute painful crises, pre-eclampsia, infection, thromboembolic events, caesarean section and hospitalization, and some studies also describe increased maternal mortality. Fetal complications include miscarriage, premature labour, fetal growth restriction and perinatal mortality.

Dehydration, cold hypoxia, overexertion, stress, and nausea and vomiting in pregnancy can precipitate crises.

2. Optimize medication and vaccinations.

   Patients with SCD are hyposplenic and at risk of infection. Penicillin prophylaxis or equivalent should be prescribed. The following vaccines are recommended:

   - *H. influenza* type b and the conjugate meningococcal C vaccine as a single dose
   - pneumococcal vaccine every five years
   - hepatitis B vaccination with immunity check
   - annual influenza vaccine

   Folic acid 5 mg daily is recommended both before conception and throughout pregnancy.

   Hydroxycarbamide, ACE inhibitors and angiotensin receptor blockers should be stopped 3 months before conception.

   Contraceptive advice should be given.

3. Assess for end-organ damage.

   - Blood pressure (BP) measurement, urinalysis, renal and liver function tests for sickle nephropathy and deranged hepatic function.
   - Retinal screening for proliferative retinopathy.
   - Screening for pulmonary hypertension with echocardiography.
   - Screening for iron overload in women who have had multiple transfusions or high ferritin levels. Some women may benefit from iron chelation prior to conception.
   - Screening for red cell antibodies that may indicate an increased risk of haemolytic disease of the newborn.

4. Offer partner testing at this point and provide counselling about prenatal diagnosis and pre-implantation genetic diagnosis if appropriate. Table 7.4.1 shows the conditions requiring counselling when the mother is affected by SCD.

Table 7.4.1 Conditions requiring counselling when the mother is affected by sickle cell disease
HbS
B-thalassaemia
HbC
D-Punjab
DB-thalassaemia
Lepore
HbE
Hereditary persistence of fetal haemoglobin (HPFH)

ANTENATAL CARE

Many women become pregnant without pre-conception care. Therefore, all the actions outlined above should take place as early as possible. Live attenuated vaccines should be deferred until after delivery. Antenatal care should be provided by a multidisciplinary team including an obstetrician with experience of high-risk antenatal care, a haematologist with an interest in SCD and a midwife.

As women with SCD are at risk of pre-eclampsia, low-dose aspirin 75 mg daily may be considered from 12 weeks of gestation.[6] Prophylactic low-molecular-weight heparin (LMWH) should be administered during antenatal hospital admission. Non-steroidal anti-inflammatory drugs (NSAIDs) should be prescribed only between 12 and 28 weeks of gestation because of potential risks to fetal development.

Blood pressure and urinalysis should be performed at each visit, and a mid-stream specimen of urine (MSU) should be sent for culture on a monthly basis.

Women with SCD should be given routine antenatal care plus additional care tailored to SCD. Ultrasound scans for fetal biometry should be done every 4 weeks from 24 weeks of gestation to monitor for intrauterine growth restriction.

Iron should only be given if there is evidence of iron deficiency.

An anaesthetic assessment should be undertaken to discuss analgesia and anaesthesia in case of operative delivery. General anaesthetic can precipitate an acute sickle crisis.

INTRAPARTUM CARE

In the absence of fetal growth restriction, it is recommended that delivery be planned from 38 weeks gestation onwards to prevent late pregnancy complications and adverse events. SCD in itself is not a contraindication to vaginal delivery. Some women may have had hip replacements because of avascular necrosis of the hip. Mode of delivery should therefore take into account any potential positional difficulties during labour or instrumental delivery.

Hospital birth is advisable, with continuous fetal heart rate monitoring in labour. The woman should be kept warm, well hydrated and well oxygenated. Pethidine should be avoided because of the risk of inducing seizures, but other opiates can be used. Regional anaesthesia is recommended for caesarean section. Indications for epidural analgesia are the same as for any other pregnant woman as per NICE intrapartum guidelines.[7]

POSTPARTUM CARE

Maintain oxygen saturation >94% and keep the woman well hydrated as the risk of sickle crisis remains elevated.

LMWH should be administered until discharge and for 7 days postpartum after a vaginal delivery, or for 6 weeks after a caesarean section.

Contraception should be discussed. Progestogen-containing contraceptives such as the progesterone-only pill, injectable contraceptives such as Depo-Provera and the levonorgestrel intrauterine system are safe and effective. The combined oral contraceptive pill is used as a second-line agent because of concern about an increased risk of thrombosis.[2]

Sickle cell crisis

NICE published guidance in June 2012 in response to variable management of acute painful sickle cell crisis throughout the UK. This was a frequent source of complaint from patients, among others such as unacceptable delays in receiving analgesia, insufficient or excessive doses, inappropriate analgesia and stigmatizing the patient as drug-seeking. The guideline includes the management of acute painful sickle cell episodes in children and young people and in pregnant women.[8]

Acute painful sickle cell crises (episodes) are caused by blockage of the small blood vessels by erythrocytes that assume a sickle shape under a variety of conditions, including dehydration, low oxygen levels and elevated temperature. However, episodes may occur unpredictably and with varying frequency from less than one episode a year to as frequent as once a week. Repeated episodes may result in organ damage. The primary goal in the management of an acute painful sickle cell episode is to achieve effective pain control both promptly and safely. A summary of recommendations is shown in Table 7.4.2. For more detail, the reader is referred to the full guidance available at www.nice.org.uk.[8]

Table 7.4.2 Summary of recommendations on the management of a sickle cell acute painful episode, incorporating NICE Clinical Guideline 143[8]

Treatment and care should take into account patients' needs and preferences. Regard patients as experts in their condition.

Treat an acute painful episode as a medical emergency.

Assess pain using a pain scoring tool. Consider pain to be severe if the score is > 7 on a visual analogue scale.

Offer analgesia within 30 minutes of presentation.

Clinical assessment should include blood pressure, pulse rate, oxygen saturation, respiratory rate, temperature.

Consider an alternative diagnosis, especially if the pain is atypical.

Offer a bolus dose of a strong opiate to all patients with severe pain or moderate pain if some analgesia has already been used. Consider a weak opiate for moderate pain if no analgesia has been used. Offer regular paracetamol. Do not offer pethidine. Reassess the need for analgesia every 30 minutes until satisfactory pain relief is achieved, and at least 4-hourly thereafter.

Consider patient-controlled analgesia (PCA).

NSAIDs should be avoided in pregnancy.

Offer regular laxatives and antiemetics and antipruritics as needed for patients taking an opiate.

Monitor the fetal heart.

Ensure adequate hydration.

Provide thromboprophylaxis.

Involve a multidisciplinary team, to include haematologist, anaesthetist, obstetrician and midwife.

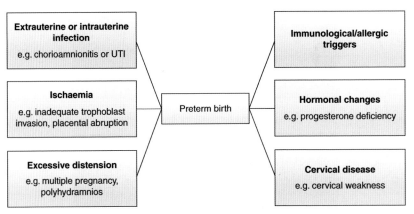

Figure 5.1 Pathological triggers of preterm birth.

(a)

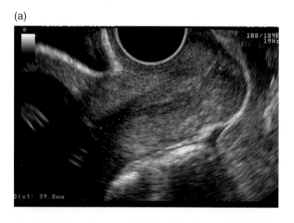

(b)

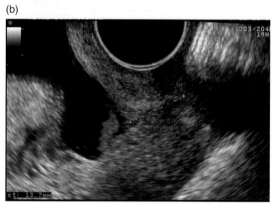

Figure 5.2 Transvaginal ultrasound illustrating (a) a normal cervical length and (b) a shortened cervix demonstrating funnelling.

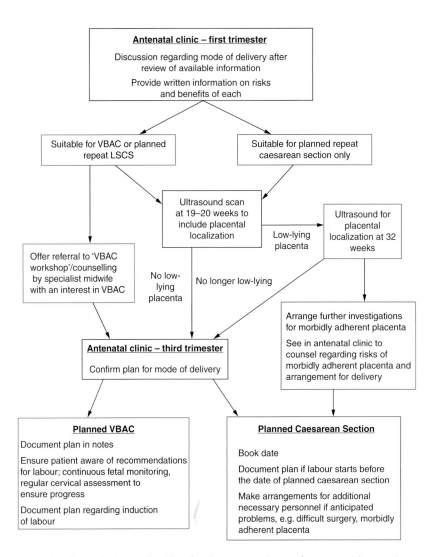

Figure 6.1 Suggested care algorithm for the antenatal care of women with a previous caesarean section.

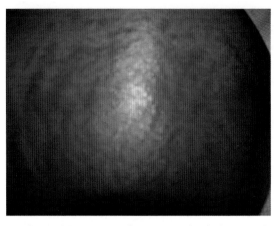

Figure 7.8.1 Polymorphic eruption of pregnancy (PEP), showing characteristic urticarial plaques in the striae with umbilical sparing (Source: WikiCommons).

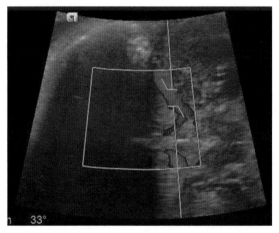

Figure 9.1 **Measurement of middle cerebral artery peak systolic velocity.** This is an ultrasound image of the fetal head, taken in transverse section at the level of the base of the skull. Colour Doppler has been used to visualize the circle of Willis, and the two middle cerebral arteries (MCAs) can be seen. The Doppler gate has been placed close to the origin of the MCA from the circle of Willis, and an angle correction has been applied to ensure a true reading of the velocity of blood flow.

Clinicians should be aware of other possible complications seen with an acute painful episode:

- acute chest syndrome
- acute stroke
- aplastic crisis
- infection
- osteomyelitis
- splenic sequestration

Thrombocytopenia

The normal platelet count in a non-pregnant woman is 140–400 × 10^9/L. Platelet counts tend to fall in normal pregnancy, particularly towards term, and although the lower limit in pregnancy is considered to be 106–120 × 10^9/L this could drop much lower. This is gestational thrombocytopenia. It is found in approximately 5% of pregnancies with no maternal or fetal sequelae. Features include mild asymptomatic thrombocytopenia, no previous history of thrombocytopenia other than in a previous pregnancy and spontaneous resolution after delivery.[9]

For descriptive purposes thrombocytopenia is divided into:

- mild thrombocytopenia (platelet count 80–140 × 10^9/L)
- moderate thrombocytopenia (platelet count 50–80 × 10^9/L)
- severe thrombocytopenia (platelet count < 50 × 10^9/L)

Table 7.4.3 shows a list of clinically important causes of maternal thrombocytopenia. Subsequent management will depend on the cause of thrombocytopenia.

Table 7.4.3   Clinically important causes of maternal thrombocytopenia

Failure of platelet production
- Bone marrow suppression due to drugs, malignancy, infection, e.g. parvovirus
- Aplastic anaemia

Platelet destruction or consumption and splenic sequestration
- Pre-eclampsia/HELLP syndrome
- Disseminated intravascular coagulation (DIC)
- Viral Infection (HIV, hepatitis C, Epstein–Barr, parvovirus, TORCH)
- Immune thrombocytopenic purpura (ITP)
- Thrombotic thrombocytopenic purpura (TTP)
- Haemolytic uraemic syndrome (HUS)
- Antiphospholipid syndrome (aPS)
- Systemic lupus erythematosus (SLE)
- Heparin-induced thrombocytopenia (HIT)
- Splenomegaly
- Myeloproliferative/lymphoproliferative disorders

Immune thrombocytopenic purpura (ITP)

This is an autoimmune condition in which antiplatelet antibodies (IgG) initiate platelet destruction, causing maternal thrombocytopenia. It is a diagnosis of exclusion after other causes of thrombocytopenia have been ruled out. IgG antibodies can cross the placenta and can cause fetal thrombocytopenia in 10% of cases. It is estimated that intracranial haemorrhage affects 2 per 100,000 births. There is poor correlation between maternal platelet count and fetal thrombocytopenia, and given the rarity of fetal sequelae from ITP, routine obstetric management in most cases is recommended.

Antenatal management of ITP depends on a number of factors, and these include the patient's previous experience with ITP, the severity of ITP and the gestational age. Serial platelet counts should be undertaken, and as long as the platelet count remains $> 100 \times 10^9$/L, this may be repeated every 4 weeks until 36 weeks of gestation and then every 2 weeks until delivery. Platelet counts $< 100 \times 10^9$/L need more frequent monitoring. Anaesthetic and paediatric alerts should be completed.

A platelet count should be checked when the patient is admitted in labour. A level $< 80 \times 10^9$/L is a contraindication for regional anaesthesia as well as fetal scalp electrode application, fetal blood sampling, ventouse delivery and rotational forceps delivery. Maternal haemorrhage is an obvious concern, but this is unlikely to occur if the platelet count is $> 50 \times 10^9$/L. In labour, active management of the third stage is recommended, as is intravenous access and a 'group and save'.

Treatment to elevate the platelet count may become necessary if the level drops to $< 50 \times 10^9$/L. This decision must be made in conjunction with a haematologist. Oral prednisolone (1 mg/kg/day) is the first line of treatment, followed by intravenous immunoglobulin (IVIG) as second-line treatment.

The decision to induce labour or to perform a caesarean section is usually made for obstetric reasons alone. A platelet count should be checked 6 weeks postpartum to ensure that it has returned to normal. If this does not occur, the general practitioner should refer the patient to a haematologist for further assessment.

At delivery, an umbilical cord blood sample should be taken to obtain a platelet count, which should also be monitored 2–5 days after delivery, as this is when a nadir is often seen.

Thrombotic thrombocytopenic purpura (TTP)

This microangiopathy is a rare condition with a reported incidence of 6 per million per year in the UK general population. The purpose of including this condition is that it is an important diagnosis to make because the untreated mortality is 90% – half of which occurs within 24 hours of presentation. This can be reduced with prompt plasma exchange.[10] Pregnancy can be the initiating event for 5–25% of cases of TTP.

Congenital and acute acquired TTP are due to a deficiency of von Willebrand factor (VWF) cleaving protein, also known as ADAMTS13. In the absence of ADAMTS13, ultra-large multimers of VWF released from the endothelium are not cleaved appropriately and cause spontaneous platelet aggregates in conditions of high shear, such as in the microvasculature of the brain, heart and kidneys.[11] Thrombosis can occur in the placenta, resulting in fetal growth restriction and fetal death.

Clinical features include microangiopathic haemolytic anaemia (MAHA) and the presence of schistocytes on a blood film, thrombocytopenia, raised BP, abdominal pain, renal impairment and neurological symptoms. The clotting screen is usually normal.

Diagnosis is difficult, owing to clinical overlap with pre-eclampsia, HELLP and haemolytic uraemic syndrome (HUS), especially if TTP occurs postpartum. While decreased ADAMTS13 activity has been reported in a wide variety of non-TTP conditions, severe ADAMTS13 deficiency ($< 5\%$) may be more helpful in distinguishing acute TTP from HUS.

Neonatal alloimmune thrombocytopenia (NAIT)

This refers to a disorder in which fetal platelets contain an antigen inherited from the father that the mother lacks. Maternal antibodies to the fetal antigens cross the placenta and bind to fetal platelets, causing fetal thrombocytopenia. The mother remains asymptomatic. Most cases in Caucasians (80%) are due to antibodies directed against platelet antigen HPA-1a. Approximately 98% of Caucasians express HPA-1a and about 2% are HPA-1a negative (HPA-1b homozygous). Ten per cent of these HPA-1a negative women will form IgG antibodies against the foreign paternal antigen. The HPA-5b antigen is the second most common cause of NAIT among Caucasians, while the HPA-4 system is the most common cause of NAIT among Asians. More than a dozen platelet antigens have been associated with NAIT, and the prevalence of these varies among different ethnic groups.

NAIT can cause intracranial haemorrhage in the first affected pregnancy (unlike rhesus alloimmunization, which develops in successive pregnancies). With each successive pregnancy, thrombocytopenia occurs at earlier gestation and tends to be more severe. NAIT should be suspected whenever a fetal intracranial haemorrhage is observed sonographically or neonatal thrombocytopenia is noted. The diagnosis is confirmed after maternal and paternal platelet typing reveals that the father has a platelet antigen that the mother lacks and the mother has detectable antibodies to this antigen.[12,13]

Antenatal management is controversial. More recently the invasive option of serial intravascular fetal platelet transfusions is being superseded by conservative therapy employing maternal intravenous immunoglobin infusions, alone or in combination with oral prednisolone therapy.

Thrombophilia

Thrombophilia is a predisposition to thrombosis. This can be inherited or acquired. Pregnancy itself is a thrombophilic state due to an increase in clotting factors and decrease in naturally occurring anticoagulants. This section gives an overview of the management of thrombophilia in pregnancy. It does not deal with the diagnosis and treatment of venous thromboembolism in pregnancy but gives a framework for managing women who have been diagnosed with a thrombophilia. The predisposition to thrombosis is not unique to laboratory-reported thrombophilia. Many other predispositions to thrombosis exist, and these are outlined in Table 7.4.4.

There are approximately 700,000 births per year in the UK, and with an estimate of the incidence of venous thromboembolism (VTE) in pregnancy and the puerperium of 1–2 per 1000, this translates into 700–1400 cases of pregnancy-related VTE per year. The overall case fatality rate for VTE in pregnancy is estimated to be 1%.[14] NICE estimates that LMWH reduces the risk of VTE in medical and surgical patients by 60–70%. Caesarean section is a risk, but women who deliver vaginally may also be at risk and this must not be overlooked. The risk is particularly increased in the postpartum period, but many antenatal VTE events occur in the first trimester, and if thromboprophylaxis is indicated it should begin early in pregnancy.

Patients may have a diagnosis of an acquired or inherited thrombophilia made following investigations for adverse pregnancy outcome, criteria for which are detailed in Table 7.4.5, or a diagnosis of thrombosis, or after family screening. It is prudent to obtain a thrombosis history to be able to decide on whether thromboprophylaxis is indicated and the length of thromboprophylaxis. All

Table 7.4.4   Some risk factors for thrombosis (not an exhaustive list)
Age > 35 years
BMI > 30 (BMI > 40 is considered as two risk factors)
Parity ≥ 3
Smoker
Personal or family history of venous thromboembolism (VTE)
Multiple pregnancy or assisted reproductive therapies
Hyperemesis/ovarian hyperstimulation syndrome
Comorbidities (e.g. heart or lung disease, inflammatory conditions, malignancy, sickle cell disease)
Pre-eclampsia
Gross varicose veins
Hospital admission or long-distance travel or immobility
Prolonged labour (> 24 hours)
Postpartum haemorrhage (> 1 litre or blood transfusion)
Operative delivery (caesarean section or mid-cavity rotational instrumental delivery)

Table 7.4.5 Obstetric criteria for the diagnosis of primary antiphospholipid syndrome

1. One or more unexplained deaths of a morphologically normal fetus at or beyond the 10th week of gestation.

2. One or more preterm births of a morphologically normal neonate before the 34th week of gestation because of (i) eclampsia or severe pre-eclampsia or (ii) recognized features of placental insufficiency.

3. Three or more unexplained consecutive spontaneous miscarriages before the 10th week of gestation, with maternal anatomic or hormonal abnormalities and paternal and maternal chromosomal cause excluded.

The primary antiphospholipid syndrome is diagnosed when at least one clinical criterion and laboratory criteria are met.[15]

Table 7.4.6 Suggested low-molecular-weight heparin (LMWH) doses for thromboprophylaxis

Weight (kg)	Enoxaparin (mg)	Dalteparin (units)	Tinzaparin (units)
< 50	20 mg daily	2500 units daily	3500 units daily
50–90	40 mg daily	5000 units daily	4500 units daily
91–130	60 mg daily	7500 units daily	7000 units daily
131–170	80 mg daily	10000 units daily	9000 units daily
> 170	0.6mg/kg/day	75 units/kg/day	75 units/kg/day
Treatment dose	1 mg/kg 12 hourly if antenatal, or 1.5 mg/kg if postnatal	100 units/kg 12 hourly if antenatal, or 200 units/kg/day if postnatal	175 units/kg/day antenatal or postnatal

In unwell women or renal patients, check estimated glomerular filtration rate (eGFR) and reduce dose accordingly. For women weighing > 90 kg, LMWH may be given in divided doses.[14]

women should undergo a risk assessment for VTE early in pregnancy and on admission to hospital or if any intercurrent problem develops. The usual type of thromboprophylaxis used is any formulation of LMWH, because of its safety and ease of use compared with unfractionated heparin. The dosage used depends on the patient's weight. If thromboprophylaxis is indicated, graduated compression stockings (GCS) should be advised for daytime wear also. The dose conversion for various types of LMWH is shown in Table 7.4.6. This table also shows a suggested dosage regime based on the woman's weight, adopted from the RCOG Green-top Guideline No. 37a (2009).[14] This is one such regime, and individual hospitals may have their own agreed regimes.

Women with three or more risk factors should be considered for thromboprophylaxis antenatally. Women with two or more persisting risk factors should be considered for thromboprophylaxis for at least 7 days postpartum. The length of postpartum thromboprophylaxis may be extended to 6 weeks if there is a personal or family history of thrombosis or other risk factor present. A woman who required prophylactic LMWH antenatally should usually continue this for 6 weeks postnatally. The reader is referred to RCOG Green-top Guideline No. 37a for detailed risk factors.[14] Women with antithrombin III deficiency (the most thrombogenic of all thrombophilia) or multiple inherited thrombophilia including homozygous factor V Leiden (FVL) should be managed jointly with a haematologist.

Key summary points

- An acute sickle cell painful episode should be treated as a medical emergency with the aim of achieving effective pain control both promptly and safely. Involve the haematologist sooner rather than later.

- Immune thrombocytopenic purpura (ITP) is a diagnosis of exclusion. The decision to induce labour or to perform a caesarean section is usually made for obstetric reasons alone.

- Neonatal alloimmune thrombocytopenia (NAIT) is uncommon but can cause intracranial haemorrhage and should be suspected whenever fetal intracranial haemorrhage is observed sonographically or neonatal thrombocytopenia is noted.

- There are approximately 700–1400 cases of pregnancy-related venous thromboembolism (VTE) per year in the UK.

- The overall case fatality rate for VTE in pregnancy is estimated to be 1%.

References

1. Ryan K, Bain BJ, Worthington D, et al. Significant haemoglobinopathies: guidelines for screening and diagnosis. Br J Haematol 2010; 149: 35–49.

2. Royal College of Obstetricians and Gynaecologists. Management of Sickle Cell Disease in Pregnancy. Green-top Guideline No. 61. London: RCOG, 2011.

3. Streetly A, Latinovic R, Henthorn J. Positive screening and carrier results for the England-wide universal newborn sickle cell screening programme by ethnicity and area for 2005–07. J Clin Pathol 2010; 63: 626–9.

4. Telfer P, Coen P, Chakravorty S, et al. Clinical outcomes in children with sickle cell disease living in England: a neonatal cohort in East London. Haematologica 2007; 92: 905–12.

5. NHS. NHS Sickle Cell and Thalassaemia Screening Programme. Standards for the Linked Antenatal and Newborn Screening Programme. London: UK National Screening Committee, 2011.

6. National Institute for Health and Care Excellence (NICE). Hypertension in Pregnancy: the Management of Hypertensive Disorders during Pregnancy. NICE Clinical Guideline CG107. London: NICE, 2010.

7. National Institute for Health and Care Excellence (NICE). Intrapartum Care. NICE Clinical Guideline CG55. London: NICE, 2008.

8. National Institute for Health and Care Excellence (NICE). Sickle Cell Acute Painful Episode: Management of an Acute Painful Sickle Cell Episode in Hospital. NICE Clinical Guideline CG143. London: NICE, 2012.

9. George JN, Woolf SH, Raskob GE, *et al.* Idiopathic thrombocytopenic purpura: a practice guideline developed by explicit methods for the American Society of Hematology. *Blood* 1996; 88: 3–40.

10. Scully M, Yarranton H, Liesner R, *et al.* Regional UK TTP registry: correlation with laboratory ADAMTS 13 analysis and clinical features. *Br J Haematol* 2008; 142: 819–26.

11. Scully M, Hunt BJ, Benjamin S, *et al.* Guidelines on the diagnosis and management of thrombotic thrombocytopenic purpura and other thrombotic microangiopathies. *Br J Haematol* 2012; 158: 323–35.

12. Bussel JB, Berkowitz RL, McFarland JG. Maternal IVIG in neonatal alloimmune thrombocytopenia. *Br J Haematol* 1997; 98: 493–4.

13. Kjeldsen-Kragh J, Killie MK, Tomter G, *et al.* A screening and intervention program aimed to reduce mortality and serious morbidity associated with severe neonatal alloimmune thrombocytopenia. *Blood* 2007; 110: 833–9.

14. Royal College of Obstetricians and Gynaecologists. *Reducing the Risk of Thrombosis and Embolism during Pregnancy and the Puerperium.* Green-top Guideline No. 37a. London: RCOG, 2009.

15. Keeling D, Mackie I, Moore GW, Greer IA, Greaves M. Guidelines on the investigation and management of antiphospholipid syndrome. *Br J Haematol* 2012; 157: 47–58.

7.5 MALIGNANCY

Sarah Vause

Introduction

Malignant disease in pregnancy is rare, with an incidence of approximately 1 in 1000–1500 pregnant women. The commonest malignancies encountered in pregnancy are cervical, breast, melanoma, ovarian and acute leukaemia.

One of the consensus views of the RCOG Cancer and Reproductive Health Study Group was that 'all cancer multidisciplinary teams should consider the possible consequences of cancer treatment for fertility and reproductive health.'[1] Therefore, this section will also consider pregnancy following previous treatment for cancer (or pre-invasive disease) and pregnancy in a woman who has previously had gestational trophoblastic disease.

Diagnosis of a malignancy may occur later than in the non-pregnant woman, resulting in more advanced stage of disease at diagnosis, although in general the course of the malignancy does not appear to be affected by pregnancy. The presence of cancer in itself does not affect fetal wellbeing, although the fetus may need to be delivered prematurely to facilitate commencement of maternal treatment, and the long-term health and wellbeing of the mother should be prioritized over that of the fetus.

Cervical cancer

This is the most common cancer diagnosed in pregnancy, with squamous cell carcinoma accounting for 80% of cervical cancer in pregnancy. At the time of diagnosis 70% of cervical carcinomas are FIGO stage I or IIA.

Following a cervical smear test, a woman who meets the criteria for colposcopy still needs colposcopy if she is pregnant. This should be done by an experienced colposcopist. The primary aim is to exclude invasive disease and to defer biopsy/ treatment of pre-invasive disease until the woman has delivered. If invasive disease is suspected clinically or colposcopically, a biopsy adequate to make the diagnosis is essential. Cone, wedge and diathermy loop biopsies in pregnancy are all associated with a risk of haemorrhage of approximately 25%.

Treatment of cervical cancer will depend on the staging at diagnosis and the gestation of the pregnancy. Specialist advice and intensive discussions with the woman are needed to determine the appropriate balance between early treatment and a successful pregnancy outcome. Trachelectomy may be an option, and concomitant insertion of a cervical suture may be considered. The pregnancy is subsequently at high risk and should be managed by a regional obstetric centre with level III neonatal facilities. Women with early-stage disease (FIGO IA1–IB1) diagnosed after 20 weeks of pregnancy may choose to attain fetal viability prior to treatment. For women with more advanced disease (FIGO IB2 and IIA), early surgical treatment is suggested – this may be done in conjunction with termination of pregnancy or caesarean section. There is a greater risk of haemorrhage, but the cure rates are similar to those in the non-pregnant patient. There is no difference in survival between pregnant and non-pregnant women matched for the same stage at diagnosis.

Advanced disease is treated with radiotherapy.

PREVIOUS TREATMENT

All women who have had two LLETZ or one knife conization procedures have a higher risk of preterm pre-labour rupture of membranes and preterm delivery in a subsequent pregnancy. This needs to be considered when managing their obstetric care.

Breast cancer

Survival rates in pregnant and non-pregnant women matched for age, tumour type and stage at diagnosis are identical. However, pregnant women tend to be diagnosed at a later stage, and at the time of diagnosis more than half have nodal involvement. The later diagnosis may be due to the clinical diagnosis being difficult in pregnancy because of active breast tissue, reluctance to refer for further investigation, difficulty interpreting mammograms during pregnancy, or reluctance to biopsy during pregnancy. Ultrasound-directed biopsy, mammography and MRI scan are all safe to perform during pregnancy.

Treatment of breast cancer during pregnancy will require discussion between the woman, the oncologist and the obstetrician, and will include discussions regarding future fertility. Generally the data for immediate treatment are reassuring, and delay or refusal to undergo therapy has serious consequences. Surgical treatment can be undertaken in all trimesters, although reconstructive surgery is best delayed until after pregnancy to achieve a better cosmetic effect. Radiotherapy should be avoided during pregnancy unless essential to preserve function, e.g. treatment of spinal metastasis. Chemotherapy should be deferred until after the first trimester, because of the risk of teratogenesis, but can then be commenced in the second trimester. If possible, delivery should be planned 2–3 weeks after the last chemotherapy session, to allow recovery of any chemotherapy-induced neutropenia and minimize the risk of sepsis.

Breastfeeding while undergoing chemotherapy, taking tamoxifen or trastuzumab is not advised.

Non-hormonal contraception is recommended even in women whose tumours are oestrogen receptor negative.

Following treatment for non-metastatic breast cancer, women are generally advised not to get pregnant for 2 years. In women who are oestrogen receptor positive, 5 years of tamoxifen treatment is usually recommended, and due to the long half-life of tamoxifen it is usually recommended that women do not try to conceive until 3 months after stopping tamoxifen. However, each woman would need to consider her own personal situation, age, desire for further family and possible increased risk of infertility when deciding when to start trying to conceive, and some may try sooner. Women with metastatic breast cancer should be advised not to conceive.

Subsequent pregnancy does not appear to have a deleterious effect on the risk of recurrence. Prior treatment for breast cancer does not appear to have a deleterious effect on pregnancy outcome.

Ovarian cancer

This may present with symptoms or be an incidental finding on an ultrasound scan performed in pregnancy.

Of adnexal masses seen in pregnancy:

- functional cysts 17%
- dermoid cysts 36%
- cystadenomas 27%
- malignancies 2–5%

Of the ovarian malignancies diagnosed in pregnancy, germ cell tumours and epithelial malignancies are approximately equal in number, each constituting approximately 40% of the total. The majority of the remaining 20% are gonadal stromal cell tumours. This differs from the overall pattern seen with ovarian malignancy, and reflects the younger age group of the women.

Most tumours are stage I at the time of diagnosis. This again contrasts with the overall pattern for ovarian malignancy.

CA125 and many other tumour markers are not reliable in pregnancy.

It has been suggested that masses that are larger than 6 cm, have a significant solid component, are bilateral, or persist after 14 weeks gestation should be surgically treated using a midline incision at 16–18 weeks of pregnancy.

Chemotherapy treatment can be used, if needed, during pregnancy.

Melanoma

The 5-year survival rates for melanomas diagnosed in pregnancy are identical to the rates for those of the same stage and thickness diagnosed in the non-pregnant population. However, the melanomas diagnosed in pregnancy tend to be thicker at the time of diagnosis than those in the non-pregnant population, suggesting that there may be a delay in making the diagnosis during pregnancy.

Surgery is the treatment of choice for early-stage melanomas, and sentinel node biopsy may be used for staging. Chemotherapy is not very effective and generally not given in pregnancy. The placenta should be sent for histology, as melanoma is the commonest cancer to have placental metastases.

Acute leukaemia

Pregnancy does not alter its course. The investigation is the same as in the non-pregnant woman. The main risks associated with pregnancy are bleeding and infection due to thrombocytopenia and leucopenia.

If needed, treatment should be continued during pregnancy. It is better to use a standard regime of proven efficacy and counsel about the risks to the fetus, rather than using an unproven regime of dubious efficacy which is thought to be safer for the fetus.

Chronic myeloid leukaemia, chronic lymphatic leukaemia and myeloma are rare in the childbearing age group.

Pregnancy following previous chemotherapy

Women who have received chemotherapy with anthracyclines (doxorubicin, epirubicin) may have ventricular dysfunction, and therefore should have echocardiography performed in a subsequent pregnancy.

A reduction in fertility may occur following chemotherapy, and various fertility-preserving techniques have been used. These should be discussed with women of reproductive age prior to commencing chemotherapy treatment. They are discussed more fully in the RCOG Green-top Guideline No. 12, *Pregnancy and Breast Cancer*.[2]

Gestational trophoblastic disease

It would be unusual to see a woman with a molar pregnancy in the antenatal clinic, as these usually present to the gynaecological services with irregular vaginal bleeding, hyperemesis or early failed pregnancy.

Any woman who develops persistent vaginal bleeding after a pregnancy event is at risk of having gestational trophoblastic neoplasia. Although this is most commonly seen after a molar pregnancy, it can occur after a live birth with an incidence estimated at 1 in 50,000. Again, this is not likely to be seen in the antenatal clinic.

A much more common scenario in the antenatal clinic is a woman who has had a previous molar or partial molar pregnancy. Women should have been advised not to conceive until their follow-up is complete. The risk of a further molar pregnancy is low (1 in 80) and women are not at increased risk of other obstetric complications. All women should notify the screening centre at the end of any future pregnancy, and hCG levels are measured 6–8 weeks after the end of the pregnancy to exclude disease recurrence.

A much rarer scenario which may be encountered in the antenatal clinic is a twin pregnancy combining a molar pregnancy with a viable fetus. In this situation, advice should be sought from the regional fetal medicine unit and the relevant trophoblastic screening centre. Prenatal invasive testing for fetal karyotype should be considered in cases where it is unclear if the pregnancy is a complete mole (diploid) with a coexisting normal twin or a partial mole (triploid).

The outcome for a normal pregnancy with a coexisting complete mole is poor, with approximately a 25% chance of achieving a live birth. There is an increased risk of early fetal loss (40%) and premature delivery (36%). The incidence of pre-eclampsia is variable, with rates as high as 20% reported, although figures were lower in a series from the UK. These women should be registered with the Gestational Trophoblastic Disease Screening service for follow-up.

See the RCOG Green-top Guideline No. 38, *The Management of Gestational Trophoblastic Disease*, for further information.[3]

Key summary points

- Diagnosis of a malignancy may occur later than in the non-pregnant woman, resulting in more advanced stage of disease at diagnosis.
- For many types of cancers the course of the malignancy does not appear to be affected by pregnancy.
- Women with malignant disease in pregnancy should be managed by a multidisciplinary team.
- When considering treatment, the long-term health and wellbeing of the mother should be prioritized over that of the fetus.

References

1. Kehoe S, Jauniaux E, Martin-Hirsch P, Savage P. Consensus views arising from the 55th Study Group: cancer and reproductive health. In *Cancer and Reproductive Health*. London: RCOG Press, 2008, chapter 22.

2. Royal College of Obstetricians and Gynaecologists. *Pregnancy and Breast Cancer*. Green-top Guideline No. 12. London: RCOG, 2011.

3. Royal College of Obstetricians and Gynaecologists. *The Management of Gestational Trophoblastic Disease*. Green-top Guideline No. 38. London: RCOG, 2010.

7.6 OBESITY

Shehnaaz Jivraj

The scale of the problem

In the UK, Public Health England (PHE) is an agency of the Department of Health (DoH) that was established in April 2013 to bring together scientists, researchers and public health professionals from more than 70 organizations to work under a single public health service. The first of the seven priorities published by PHE was to help people live longer and healthier lives by reducing preventable deaths and the burden of ill health associated with smoking, high blood pressure, obesity, poor diet, poor mental health, insufficient exercise and alcohol. The Public Health England Obesity Knowledge and Intelligence team (formerly the National Obesity Observatory) provides a single point of contact for information on data, evaluation, evidence and research related to weight status and its determinants. PHE obtains its obesity data from three main sources: Health Survey for England (HSE), model-based estimates using HSE, and the Quality and Outcomes Framework (QOF). The HSE is an annual survey undertaken since 1991, currently commissioned by the Health and Social Care Information Centre, and is presently the most robust data source to monitor trends in adult obesity in England.

Within the UK population, the proportion of adults with a normal body mass index (BMI) decreased between 1993 and 2011, from 41% to 34% among men and from 49% to 39% among women. Among both men and women there has been little change in the proportion that was overweight over this period (41% of men and 33% of women in 2011). However, there has been a marked increase in the proportion that is obese. This increased from 13% of men in 1993 to 24% in 2011, and from 16% of women in 1993 to 26% in 2011. More worryingly, obesity in women in 2010 and 2011 was at its highest level since 1993. Once thought to be an epidemic of the industrialized world, the problem of obesity is becoming a more global problem.

Key facts from the World Health Organization (WHO) state that worldwide obesity has nearly doubled since 1980. In 2008, 35% of adults aged 20 and older were overweight and 11% were obese. Of these, over 200 million men and nearly 300 million women were obese. It thus appears that globally (and not just the UK) obesity is more prevalent among women than men. In 2011, more than 40 million children under the age of five were overweight. Once considered a high-income-country problem, overweight and obesity are now on the rise in low- and middle-income countries, particularly in urban settings.

The fundamental cause of obesity and overweight is an energy imbalance between calories consumed and calories expended. Globally, there has been an increased intake of energy-dense foods that are high in fat and an increase in physical inactivity due to the increasingly sedentary nature of many forms of work, changing modes of transportation, and increasing urbanization. Changes in dietary and physical activity patterns are often the result of environmental and societal changes associated with development and lack of supportive policies in sectors such as health, agriculture, transport, urban planning, environment, food processing, distribution, marketing and education.

Overweight and obesity are linked to more deaths worldwide than underweight. For example, 65% of the world's population live in countries where overweight and obesity kill more people than underweight (this includes all high-income and most middle-income countries). Raised BMI (Table 7.6.1) is a major risk factor for non-communicable diseases such as:

- cardiovascular diseases (mainly heart disease and stroke), which were the leading cause of death in 2008
- diabetes
- musculoskeletal disorders (especially osteoarthritis)
- some cancers (endometrial, breast and colon)

Many low- and middle-income countries are now facing a 'double burden' of disease. While they continue to deal with the problems of infectious disease and

Table 7.6.1 BMI definition and range. (NHS Commissioning Board. Clinical commissioning policy: complex and specialized obesity surgery)

BMI definition	BMI range (kg/m^2)
Underweight	Under 18.5
Normal	18.5 to less than 25
Overweight	25 to less than 30
Obese	30 to less than 40
Obese grade I	30 to less than 35
Obese grade II	35 to less than 40
Morbidly obese / obese grade III / severe	40 and over

undernutrition, they are experiencing a rapid upsurge in non-communicable disease risk factors such as obesity and overweight, particularly in urban settings. It is not uncommon to find undernutrition and obesity existing side by side within the same country, the same community and the same household.

Children in low- and middle-income countries are more vulnerable to inadequate prenatal, infant and young-child nutrition. At the same time, they are exposed to high-fat, high-sugar, high-salt, energy-dense, micronutrient-poor foods, which tend to be lower in cost but also lower in nutrient quality. These dietary patterns, in conjunction with lower levels of physical activity, result in sharp increases in childhood obesity, while undernutrition issues remain unsolved. Childhood obesity is associated with a higher chance of obesity, premature death and disability in adulthood. But in addition to increased future risks, obese children experience breathing difficulties, increased risk of fractures, hypertension, early markers of cardiovascular disease, insulin resistance and psychological effects. More than 30 million overweight children are living in developing countries and 10 million in developed countries.[1]

Pre-pregnancy counselling

As obstetricians, we have access to managing obesity in a window of opportunity during a woman's reproductive years. Ideally, we should provide pre-pregnancy counselling to all women who have a BMI $\geq$ 30. Unfortunately, however, many pregnancies are unplanned and this opportunity is not available. Pregnancy-related risks associated with obesity are shown in Table 7.6.2. The purpose of pre-pregnancy counselling is to inform the woman of her pregnancy-related risks associated with obesity, taking into account her previous obstetric history and any other coincidental comorbidity, and to advise her on how these risks may be reduced, including weight optimization prior to pregnancy. In addition, all women with a BMI $\geq$ 30 should be advised to take 5 mg of folic acid daily starting at least

Table 7.6.2 Obstetric risks associated with obesity
Subfertility
First-trimester miscarriage
Fetal congenital malformations
Gestational diabetes
Hypertensive disorders of pregnancy
Macrosomia
Stillbirth
Prolonged labour and postpartum haemorrhage
Caesarean section
Anaesthetic complications
Perioperative infections

1 month before conception. This recommendation is based on the premise that individuals at risk of fetal neural tube defects (NTD) should be advised to have a higher dose of folic acid. The current DoH recommendation is that all women should have folic acid 400 μg once daily until 12 weeks of gestation. Women with a raised BMI are at increased risk of fetal NTD[2] and also have lower serum folate levels,[3] which puts them at higher risk of NTDs than the general population. Women with BMI ≥ 30 should also be advised to take 10 μg of vitamin D supplementation daily during pregnancy and while breastfeeding, as they are at increased risk of vitamin D deficiency compared to women with a normal BMI.[4]

Antenatal care

Obese pregnant women are at increased risk of anaesthesia-related complications such as failure of epidural cannulation and aspiration of gastric contents under general anaesthesia. Pregnant women with a booking BMI ≥ 40 should therefore have an antenatal consultation with an obstetric anaesthetist to identify and address any potential difficulties with venous access and regional or general anaesthesia. In the third trimester, re-measurement of weight should be undertaken and any manual handling requirements for childbirth such as lateral transfer equipment, hoists, safe working loads of beds and operating tables, as well as provision of adequately sized thromboembolic deterrent (compression) stockings, should be addressed.

Maternal obesity is associated with an increased risk of deep vein thrombosis and pulmonary embolism. Thromboprophylaxis should be provided in accordance with the RCOG Clinical Green-top Guideline No. 37a.[5]

BMI ≥ 35 is a risk factor for pre-eclampsia, and this should be taken into account when assessing the risk of pre-eclampsia for recommending low-dose aspirin from 12 weeks gestation.[6]

All pregnant women with a BMI ≥ 30 should be screened for gestational diabetes with a glucose tolerance test (GTT) at 24–28 weeks. If found to have gestational diabetes, management should be in conjunction with a diabetes physician, and a postnatal GTT should be arranged at 6 weeks. Among obese non-diabetics, weight loss of at least 4.5 kg between the first and second pregnancies reduced the risk of developing gestational diabetes by up to 40% in one study.[7]

Intrapartum care

The intrapartum risks of obesity include shoulder dystocia and postpartum haemorrhage. Immediate obstetric intervention is vital in these situations. Babies born to obese mothers are more likely to require neonatal intensive care than those born to normal-weight women. In light of these observations, it is recommended that women with a BMI of ≥ 35 should give birth in a consultant-led unit with appropriate neonatal services. Active management of the third stage of labour is recommended, to reduce the risk of postpartum haemorrhage.

As venous access can be difficult, it is recommended that women with a BMI ≥ 40 should have venous access established early in labour, to avoid a difficult attempt for the first time in an emergency situation.

Operative vaginal delivery and caesarean section are often technically difficult, and appropriately experienced obstetric and anaesthetic clinicians should be present to perform or supervise delivery. As there is a higher risk of infection, antibiotics should be administered appropriately, and at caesarean section it is advisable to suture subcutaneous fat which is ≥ 2 cm deep.

Postnatal care

Obesity is associated with low breastfeeding initiation and maintenance rates, and extra specialist breastfeeding support should be provided.

Non-diabetic women should have regular follow-ups with the general practitioner (GP) to screen for the development of type 2 diabetes, and an annual screen for cardiometabolic risk factors.

A number of large randomized controlled trials (RCTs) have shown that lifestyle interventions such as exercise plus diet interventions can prevent or delay the development of diabetes in individuals with impaired glucose tolerance or the metabolic syndrome.[8]

The postnatal period is an opportunity to influence women's health in the long term, to empower and encourage them to influence their own health destinies. This is best done in conjunction with the woman's GP. Nutritional advice from appropriately trained professionals should be factored into general postnatal care.

The future

The UK has the second highest prevalence of obesity in the world. In 2013 the Royal College of Physicians (London) published a report of a working party calling for multidisciplinary input into obesity management, highlighting the role of the GP in weight management, the need for leadership in the area, including increased education and training of healthcare professionals, and even suggested that obesity should be made into a subspecialty in its own right.[9] There is no shortage of data and reports on this growing problem – the time has now come for coordinated action to tackle the problem.

Key summary points

- In the UK, the prevalence of obesity among women has increased from 16% in 1993 to 26% in 2011
- Obesity, once thought to be a disease of the developed world, is now a global problem and also affects children
- Antenatal risks include pre-eclampsia, deep vein thrombosis and gestational diabetes

- Intrapartum risks include shoulder dystocia, increased operative delivery and postpartum haemorrhage
- The postnatal period is an opportunity to influence women's health in the long term, through multidisciplinary coordinated efforts

References

1. WHO. *Obesity and Overweight.* Fact Sheet no. 311. Geneva: World Health Organization, 2013.

2. Rasmussen SA, Chu SY, Kim SY, Schmid CH, Lau J. Maternal obesity and risk of neural tube defects: a metaanalysis. *Am J Obstet Gynecol* 2008; 198: 611–19.

3. Mojtabai R. Body mass index and serum folate in childbearing age women. *Eur J Epidemiol* 2004; 19: 1029–36.

4. Centre for Maternal and Child Enquiries; Royal College of Obstetricians and Gynaecologists. *Management of Women with Obesity in Pregnancy.* CMACE/RCOG Joint Guideline. London: CMACE/RCOG, 2010.

5. Royal College of Obstetricians and Gynaecologists. *Reducing the Risk of Thrombosis and Embolism during Pregnancy and the Puerperium.* Green-top Guideline No. 37a. London: RCOG, 2009.

6. National Institute for Health and Care Excellence (NICE). *Hypertension in Pregnancy: the Management of Hypertensive Disorders during Pregnancy.* NICE Clinical Guideline CG107. London: NICE, 2010.

7. Glazer NL, Hendrickson AF, Schellenbaum GD, Mueller BA. Weight change and the risk of gestational diabetes in obese women. *Epidemiology* 2004; 15: 733–7.

8. Orozco LJ, Buchleitner AM, Gimenez-Perez G, *et al.* Exercise or exercise and diet for preventing type 2 diabetes mellitus. *Cochrane Database Syst Rev* 2008; (3): CD003054.

9. Royal College of Physicians. *Action on Obesity: Comprehensive Care for All. Report of a Working Party.* London: RCP, 2013.

7.7 KIDNEY DISEASE

Remon Keriakos

Physiological changes in renal function with pregnancy

Pregnancy dilatations of the urinary collecting system are more marked on the right-hand side, where the dilatation seen in the ureter can mimic obstructive uropathy. Bacteriuria is more likely to occur during pregnancy because of the dilated collecting system, delayed emptying, urinary stasis, and vesicoureteral reflux, and these can evolve into pyelonephritis in about one-third of cases. Acute pyelonephritis most commonly occurs during the second trimester, with the predominant pathogenic organism being *Escherichia coli.*

Renal plasma flow increases by 50–70% in pregnancy; this change is most pronounced in the first two trimesters and declines slightly in the third trimester. Glomerular filtration rate and creatinine clearance increases by 50% and is associated with a reduction in serum creatinine and urea concentrations. Renal protein excretion increases during pregnancy.[1,2] Up to 300 mg of total protein may be excreted in the urine of healthy women in 24 hours. There is a degree of water and sodium retention, and the majority of women experience some oedema. The blood pressure falls by approximately 10 mmHg in the first 24 weeks of pregnancy and gradually returns to a pre-pregnancy level by term.

Pregnancies in women with underlying chronic kidney disease, and in those who require dialysis during pregnancy or who have previously undergone renal transplantation, pose unique sets of challenges. Understanding the physiologic changes forms the basis of appropriate management of these unusual disorders.

Effect of chronic kidney disease on pregnancy

There is an increased risk of pre-eclampsia, which can be difficult to identify in women with pre-existing proteinuria and hypertension. There is also risk of intrauterine growth restriction and preterm labour. Iatrogenic preterm delivery in maternal or fetal interest is common.[2]

Effect of pregnancy on chronic kidney disease

In connective tissue disorders such as scleroderma, systemic lupus erythematosus (SLE) and polyarteritis nodosa, renal function may deteriorate rapidly. Pregnancy may be best avoided in these conditions.[3] Pregnancy increases the risk of kidney infection, which could lead to deterioration of renal function.

Women on dialysis and with transplant

Women on long-term haemodialysis or chronic ambulatory peritoneal dialysis have impaired fertility, and conception is not common. Following renal transplantation, normal endocrine function is often restored rapidly. It is not uncommon for women to become pregnant soon after renal transplantation. Women on dialysis and even those who have had transplant have a high rate of miscarriage and pregnancy complications such as intrauterine growth restriction or pre-eclampsia. If transplant recipients do wish to become pregnant they should ideally wait 2 years after the transplantation to allow graft function to stabilize. Pregnancy does not appear to alter the long-term prognosis for the mother.

Management

PRE-PREGNANCY

Pre-pregnancy counselling is essential to discuss the implications of the pregnancy on the kidney disease and associated pregnancy complications and, where possible, modification of remediable risk factors, including consideration of familial conditions and optimization of medication. Counsellors should take into account the patient's overall prognosis. Many patients with severe renal compromise and underlying disorders may themselves have a limited prognosis with regard to their health and their life. They must be aware that, should severe problems arise, termination of pregnancy may be required.

ANTEPARTUM

Women with mild renal impairment (serum creatinine < 125 mmol/L) tend to have a good outcome, whereas those with moderate (creatinine 125–275 mmol/L) to severe (creatinine > 275 mmol/L) impairment have a higher incidence of problems.[1]

Women with ≥ 1+ dipstick positive proteinuria (in the absence of infection) should have this quantified. Persistent proteinuria (> 500 mg/day) diagnosed before 20 weeks of gestation should prompt referral to a nephrologist.

When proteinuria worsens but blood pressure remains normal or easily controlled and overall renal function is stable or minimally affected, the pregnancy can be allowed to continue with suitable monitoring.

Women with moderate to severe renal dysfunction must be warned of the risk of deterioration in their renal function.

Early dialysis is necessary in pregnant women when renal function deteriorates and should be considered when the serum creatinine reaches 309 mmol/L. Longer, more frequent dialysis (20 hours/week) is associated with the best fetal outcome. Haemodialysis may therefore be necessary at least 5 days per week.

If pregnancy occurs in women on dialysis or after kidney transplant, collaboration between renal physicians and an obstetrician with a special interest in medical disorders or renal problems in pregnancy is essential. Renal function should be assessed regularly with creatinine clearance, quantitative proteinuria and serum biochemistry.[2]

Low-dose aspirin should be offered as prophylaxis against pre-eclampsia, commencing within the first trimester particularly in patients with an underlying connective tissue problem such as SLE. The decision to use aspirin in patients with moderate to severe renal problems should involve the nephrologist, as chronic inhibition of prostaglandin synthesis in the kidneys may occur.

Multidisciplinary antenatal visits should be frequent, possibly every 2 weeks till 28 weeks and then weekly thereafter.

A significant decline in renal function often triggers preterm delivery.

Blood pressure must be monitored carefully and hypertension treated. The target blood pressure should be below 140/90 mmHg.

Pre-eclampsia is difficult to diagnose in these women, since their biochemistry may be abnormal and proteinuria and hypertension already present. Optimum control of blood pressure must occur.

Proteinuria constitutes a risk for venous thromboembolism, and thromboprophylaxis should be considered.

Women should be regularly screened for urinary tract infection and promptly treated to reduce the risk of deteriorating renal function. Antibiotic prophylaxis should be given to women with recurrent bacteriuria/urinary tract infections.

Fetal growth and wellbeing should be monitored regularly.

Anaemia associated with renal compromise will require treatment with haematinics and may require transfusion or recombinant erythropoietin.

POSTPARTUM

Following delivery, renal function can deteriorate. It is important to monitor renal function and control of blood pressure following delivery. Blood pressure control can be achieved with adrenoceptor antagonists, calcium channel blockers and methyldopa.

Key summary points

- Prior to pregnancy, patients with chronic kidney disease (CKD) should receive careful pre-conception assessment and counselling.

- Multidisciplinary teams of renal physicians, obstetricians and midwifery staff enable the provision of optimal care to pregnant CKD patients.

- During pregnancy, renal function, proteinuria, blood pressure and fetal growth should be serially assessed.

- It is essential to treat infection and anaemia promptly and aggressively.

- Aspirin therapy and thromboprophylaxis should be considered.

- The decision regarding when to resort to dialysis and when to deliver the baby requires input from professionals with the relevant experience and skills.

References

1. Davison JM, Nelson-Piercy C, Kehoe S, Baker P. Consensus views arising from the 54th Study Group: renal disease in pregnancy. In *Renal Disease in Pregnancy*. London: RCOG Press, 2008, chapter 20.

2. Krane NK. Renal disease and pregnancy. *Medscape* 2013. http://emedicine.medscape.com/article/246123-overview (accessed 4 October 2015).

3. Hou S. Pregnancy in chronic renal insufficiency and end-stage renal disease. *Am J Kidney Dis* 1999; 33: 235–52.

7.8 SKIN DISORDERS

Frances Hills

Introduction

Dermatological conditions are some of the commonest chronic medical problems. Skin problems may be affected by pregnancy, or the management may need to be reviewed as a result of pregnancy. Women should be managed in conjunction with their general practitioner (GP) or dermatologist.

In addition, women may present to maternity services with new skin changes. Many are physiological in pregnancy, but there are some dermatoses that are specific to pregnancy. It is important, therefore, to be able to recognize pregnancy dermatoses and differentiate them from normal skin changes.

It is important to also consider the psychological effects on the woman from visible disease.

Physiological changes in pregnancy

Up to 90% of women experience hyperpigmentation; it is commonest in dark-skinned women. The commonest affected areas are the skin of the anterior abdomen (the linea nigra), nipples and areolae. Scars, freckles and naevi often darken. Many women develop melasma, a symmetrical macular hyperpigmentation of the face.

Striae distensae are common, particularly on the abdomen, breasts, buttocks and thighs. The initial red colour fades with time to become flesh-coloured or pale.

Hirsutism is frequent in pregnancy, due to increased production of ovarian androgens. Scalp hair thickens, and the skin may develop a furry appearance due to short lanugo hairs. This disappears postpartum.

Nail changes, such as brittleness, faster growth or grooves, are common. The vascular changes in pregnancy may lead to palmar erythema and development of spider naevi.[1]

Atopic eruption of pregnancy (AEP)

AEP is the commonest dermatosis in pregnancy, encompassing exacerbation of pre-existing atopic eczema (about 20% of cases) and new atopic skin manifestations (about 80% of cases) (Table 7.8.1).

Eczema is a chronic itchy dermatitis affecting up to 10% of the adult population. It characteristically involves flexural surfaces, such as behind the knee or in the elbow crease, but may be generalized. Affected individuals often have dry skin and a personal or family history of atopic illnesses. Complications include infection, sleep disturbance due to itching, and social or psychological problems. More than half of women experience exacerbations during pregnancy.

Women developing new atopic skin changes often have a family history of atopy. They may have typical patchy eczematous changes or papular lesions. Skin dryness is common. Total serum IgE is elevated in 20–70% of women. Normal serum bile acids help differentiate between AEP and obstetric cholestasis.[1,2]

Women should be advised to apply an emollient at least 3–4 times a day, and may also use it in the shower or bath; additives such as urea and menthol are considered to be safe.

Topical corticosteroids are considered to be safe in pregnancy, but should be used at the lowest possible potency for the shortest time necessary to control symptoms.

Oral antihistamines, such as chlorphenamine, may be used intermittently to help reduce itching and scratching, particularly at night. Secondary bacterial infections should be managed with systemic or topical antibiotics.

Systemic corticosteroids, such as prednisolone, do not cause concern if used for a few days for an acute exacerbation. Longer-term corticosteroid use or immuno-suppressive agents such as ciclosporin or azathioprine should be avoided if possible but may be necessary in severe cases.[1,3]

Polymorphic eruption of pregnancy (PEP)

PEP is also known as pruritic urticarial papules and plaques of pregnancy (PUPPP). It is a common pregnancy-specific dermatosis, occurring in about 1 in 160 pregnancies, usually beginning after 36 weeks of gestation (Table 7.8.1). It starts on the abdomen, often in the striae, as intensely itchy urticarial papules and plaques that spread to the buttocks and thighs, with periumbilical sparing. In later disease the rash may become generalized and polymorphic, including vesicles, bullae, eczematous lesions, target lesions and erythema (Figure 7.8.1).

PEP is related to abdominal distension and is commoner in primigravidae, multiple pregnancies and those with excessive weight gain. It is self-limiting, has no adverse effects on the developing fetus, and tends not to recur in future pregnancies.

Direct immunofluorescence of skin biopsy is negative.

Treatment is for symptom control. Emollients, with additives such as menthol or urea, should be used liberally. Topical corticosteroids may also be used, as can oral chlorphenamine. In severe cases a short course of oral prednisolone with a tapering dose may be used.[1,2]

Pemphigoid gestationis (PG)

PG is an autoimmune disorder occurring in 1 in 2000 to 1 in 60,000 pregnancies. It is commoner in women with HLA DR3 and DR4 haplotypes and is associated with other autoimmune disorders.

PG generally presents in the second or third trimester (Table 7.8.1). Initially there are pruritic urticarial papules and plaques. Unlike PEP, it often begins in the

Table 7.8.1 Comparison of pregnancy dermatoses

	AEP	PEP	PG
Onset	75% before 3rd trimester	Late 3rd trimester	2nd or 3rd trimester
Lesions	Eczematous or papular lesions	Papulo-urticarial rash on abdomen with periumbilical sparing Later polymorphic features	Papulo-urticarial or bullous rash on abdomen with periumbilical involvement Palms and soles
Laboratory tests	Elevated total serum IgE (20–70%) Direct immunofluorescence (DIF) negative	DIF negative	DIF positive Indirect immunofluorescence may be positive
Complications	Maternal discomfort	Maternal discomfort	Postpartum flare Neonatal lesions Small-for-dates infant
Treatment	Emollients Topical corticosteroids Oral antihistamines	Emollients Topical corticosteroids Oral antihistamines	Emollients Oral antihistamines Topical corticosteroids Systemic corticosteroids Plasmapheresis Immunosuppressive therapy

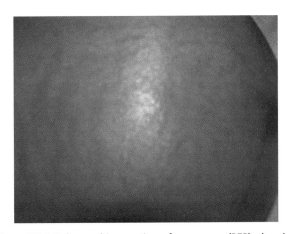

Figure 7.8.1 Polymorphic eruption of pregnancy (PEP), showing characteristic urticarial plaques in the striae with umbilical sparing (Source: WikiCommons). A black and white version of this figure will appear in some formats. For the colour version, please refer to the plate section.

periumbilical region and may spread to the abdomen, thighs, palms and soles. The face and oral mucosa are usually spared. Bullae develop within days or weeks.

PG commonly flares after delivery, and may take months or years to resolve. Menstrual flares are frequent, and recurrence in future pregnancy is usual. There is a small increase in the incidence of small-for-dates infants. Between 5% and 10% of infants have cutaneous lesions, which resolve within weeks and have no long-term sequelae.

Skin biopsy is recommended. Histology shows the presence of eosinophils and sub-epidermal blistering. Direct immunofluorescence is positive. Indirect immuno-fluorescence of serum may be positive for circulating autoantibodies.

At the pre-bullous stage, PG is managed with emollients, oral antihistamines and topical corticosteroids. In the bullous stage high-dose systemic corticosteroids are used, tapering the dose as control is achieved. The dose should be increased immediately after delivery to reduce postpartum flare.

In severe cases plasmapharesis or immunosuppressive therapy should be considered.[1,2]

Key summary points

- Atopic eruption of pregnancy (AEP) is the commonest pregnancy dermatosis, encompassing women with pre-existing eczema and women with new atopic skin disease.

- Polymorphic eruption of pregnancy (PEP) is common, has a variety of lesions including bullae, and usually spares the periumbilical region.

- Pemphigoid gestationis (PG) is rare, has a wide variety of lesions including bullae, and usually involves the periumbilical region.

- Skin biopsy with direct immunofluorescence is recommended to differentiate PG from PEP.

- Liberal use of emollients is recommended. Topical corticosteroids are considered to be safe; systemic corticosteroids may also be necessary.

References

1. Ambros-Rudolph CM. Dermatoses of pregnancy: clues to diagnosis, fetal risk and therapy. *Ann Dermatol* 2011; 23: 265–75.

2. Beard MP, Millington GW. Recent developments in the specific dermatoses of pregnancy. *Clin Exp Dermatol* 2012; 37: 1–5.

3. Primary Care Dermatology Society; British Association of Dermatologists. Guidelines for the management of atopic eczema. *Skin* 2009; 39: 399–402.

8 Cardiac disease in pregnancy

Chibuike Iruloh

Introduction

The management of cardiac disease in pregnancy is important, as there are significant risks of maternal and fetal morbidity and mortality from cardiac diseases. In the 2006–08 triennium, cardiac disease was the leading cause of death with 53 deaths (2.31 per 100,000 maternities).[1] These were the highest number and rate of cardiac deaths in pregnancy since the 1985–87 period, with increases recorded in the last three triennia. Fifty-one per cent of these deaths had sub-standard care, and most had acquired heart disease such as myocardial infarction and ischaemic heart disease, aortic dissection and cardiomyopathy.

There are significant cardiovascular changes in pregnancy which can strain the heart and mimic symptoms of cardiac disease. There is a 40% increase in cardiac output, which is due to a 25% increase in both stroke volume and heart rate. This is accompanied by a 1250–1500 mL increase in blood volume due to a 40–50% increase in plasma volume and 20% increase in red cell mass. There is a reduction in total peripheral resistance but no change in the cardiac venous pressure of the superior vena cava circulation. There is a fall in blood pressure up to 20 weeks gestation and then it gradually returns to pre-pregnancy levels by term. Cardiac output increases to 8 L/minute in the first stage of labour and 9 L/minute in the second stage. It increases by 60–80% immediately after delivery but returns to pre-labour levels within 1 hour of delivery. By 3 months postpartum cardiac output, stroke volume and peripheral vascular resistance have returned to pre-pregnancy levels. The hyperdynamic circulation of pregnancy can lead to innocent cardiac murmurs in pregnancy.

Principles of management

The management of pregnant women with cardiac diseases must be by a multi-disciplinary team comprising an obstetrician, a cardiologist with experience of

Antenatal Disorders for the MRCOG and Beyond, Second Edition, ed. Dilly Anumba and Shehnaaz Jivraj. Published by Cambridge University Press. © Cambridge University Press 2016.

cardiac disorders in pregnancy, an obstetric anaesthetist, a specialist midwife and a haematologist (for those at high risk of thromboembolism, such as women with mechanical heart valves). Those with congenital heart disease should have fetal echocardiography by a fetal cardiologist at 19–22 weeks because of the increased risk of congenital heart disease in the fetus.

All pregnant women recently arrived in the UK should have a cardiovascular assessment in primary/secondary care. Those with already diagnosed disease should have pre-conception assessment and counselling in order to assess disease status, discuss pregnancy risks and management and optimize disease state and medication (and/or contraception) prior to attempting to conceive. The patients are then seen in the first trimester (along with those with new presentations), when a plan of care is made. They should be seen regularly thereafter and a decision taken at about 32–34 weeks regarding timing, place and mode of delivery, and care during delivery and thereafter.[2] Although cardiac disease may deteriorate in the late second and third trimester, the greatest risk is at delivery and in the post-partum period when raised blood pressure and sudden changes in cardiac output and blood volume secondary to uterine contractions, vasodilatation and haemorrhage place additional strain on the heart. The aim is to minimize these changes.

A thorough history and clinical examination should be undertaken, and usually an ECG, echocardiogram and pulse oximetry would be required. Holter (24-hour) ECG or longer is useful in arrhythmias and palpitations. Other investigations that might become necessary include exercise testing, cardiac MRI and chest x-ray.

The risk associated with pregnancy is determined by the type of cardiac disease, the presence of cyanosis and pulmonary hypertension, and is often assessed using risk stratification tools such as the New York Heart Association (NYHA) classification of heart disease (Table 8.1), the World Health Organization (WHO) classification of maternal cardiovascular risk (Table 8.2) and the Cardiac Disease in Pregnancy (CARPREG) risk score. The last of these uses the presence of four groups of risk factors to predict maternal risk. The risk factors are (1) prior cardiac event such as heart failure, stroke, arrhythmia or transient ischaemic attack; (2) baseline NYHA functional class > II or cyanosis; (3) left heart obstruction (mitral valve area < 2 cm^2, aortic valve area < 1.5 cm^2, peak LV outflow tract gradient > 30 mmHg by echocardiography); and (4) reduced systemic ventricular

Table 8.1 NYHA functional classification of heart disease

Class	Symptoms
I	No breathlessness / uncompromised
II	Breathlessness on severe exertion / slightly compromised
III	Breathlessness on mild exertion / moderately compromised
IV	Breathlessness at rest / severely compromised

Table 8.2 Modified WHO classification of maternal cardiovascular risk

Class	Pregnancy risk	Conditions
I	No detectable increased risk of maternal mortality and no/mild increase in morbidity.	Uncomplicated pulmonary stenosis, PDA, mitral valve prolapse, successfully repaired ASD, VSD, PDA, atrial or ventricular ectopic beats.
II	Small increased risk of maternal mortality or moderate increase in morbidity.	Unoperated, uncomplicated VSD, ASD; repaired tetralogy of Fallot; most arrhythmias.
II-III		Mild left ventricular impairment, hypertrophic cardiomyopathy, tissue valve replacements, Marfan's syndrome with no aortic dilatation.
III	Significantly increased risk of maternal mortality or severe morbidity. Expert counselling required. If pregnancy is decided upon, intensive specialist cardiac and obstetric monitoring needed throughout pregnancy, childbirth and the puerperium.	Mechanical heart valves, systemic right heart, Fontan circulation, cyanotic heart disease, Marfan's syndrome with aortic diameter 40–45 mm.
IV	Extremely high risk of maternal mortality or severe morbidity. Pregnancy contraindicated. If pregnancy occurs, termination should be discussed. If pregnancy continues, care as for class III.	Pulmonary hypertension, severe left heart dysfunction, severe mitral stenosis, severe symptomatic aortic stenosis, Marfan's syndrome with aortic diameter > 45 mm, previous peripartum cardiomyopathy with residual left heart impairment, severe aortic coarctation.

ASD, atrial septal defect; PDA, patent ductus arteriosus; VSD, ventricular septal defect.

systolic function (ejection fraction < 40%). For each risk factor present, a point is assigned, with a 5% maternal risk if 0 point, 27% if 1 point and 75% if > 1.

Most patients would be suitable for vaginal delivery, with caesarean section reserved for obstetric reasons. Patients with acute or chronic aortic dissection, Marfan's syndrome with aortic diameter > 45 mm and intractable acute heart failure should be considered for caesarean section, while those with severe aortic stenosis, severe forms of pulmonary hypertension and acute heart failure might benefit from caesarean delivery. If labour induction is required, amniotomy and oxytocin is preferable to the use of prostaglandins. Lumbar epidural analgesia is recommended to reduce pain-related elevation in sympathetic activity and the urge to push, and to provide adequate analgesia for surgery. Continuous epidural or spinal anaesthesia can be safely used while taking into consideration the risk of hypotension, especially in patients with obstructive heart lesions. Adequate haemodynamic monitoring is necessary, with strict fluid monitoring. The second stage and the associated haemodynamic changes can be shortened by forceps or ventouse-assisted delivery. Slow oxytocin infusion in the third stage is preferred to ergometrine to minimize blood loss while avoiding the vasoconstriction and hypertension of the latter. Operative delivery must be carried out by an experienced clinician, with meticulous attention to haemostasis to minimize blood loss. Haemodynamic monitoring for at least 24 hours postpartum should be continued because of the fluid shifts during this period. Adequate thromboprophylaxis should be instituted.

Specific heart diseases

Valvular heart disease can be acquired or congenital. Rheumatic heart disease is a major problem in developing countries and in immigrants to developed countries. In the developed countries the majority of valvular lesions are congenital. Stenotic valve diseases have a higher pregnancy risk than regurgitant lesions, and left-sided lesions have a higher complication rate than right-sided diseases. There is a risk of arrhythmia with valvular heart disease. Patients with moderate or severe mitral stenosis, and symptomatic patients with severe aortic stenosis or impaired left ventricular function should be counselled against pregnancy until surgical correction has been undertaken. Medical therapy includes rest, therapy with β1-selective blockers, diuretics and anticoagulation (for arrhythmias). Percutaneous surgery is reserved for severe cases that do not improve despite optimal medical therapy. Bioprosthetic heart valves not associated with any dysfunction are generally well tolerated in pregnancy, but there is a higher risk that they will require replacement long-term. Mechanical valves have excellent performance and long-term durability but there is a high risk of thromboembolism requiring anticoagulation. Warfarin (and other oral anticoagulants) is the most effective prophylaxis against thromboembolism. However, warfarin is a dose-dependent embryotoxin (> 5 mg daily) and its use increases the risk of maternal and fetal bleeding in labour. The preferred regimen (especially if warfarin dose required exceeds 5 mg) is continuation of warfarin until conception, heparin (with anti-Xa monitoring) from 6 to 12 weeks gestation, then warfarin until late third trimester when heparin is recommenced and continued through labour (stopping at commencement of second stage).[3] Warfarin is not expressed in breastmilk.

Most palpitations are benign, but new-onset ventricular tachycardia should be investigated to exclude underlying structural heart disease. Ventricular and supraventricular arrhythmias needing treatment arise in 15% of patients with congenital heart disease. Supraventricular tachycardia can be terminated by vagal manoeuvres or intravenous adenosine if digoxin fails. Selective β-blockers may be used prophylactically if symptoms are intolerable or haemodynamic compromise exists. Pharmacological termination of atrial flutter and fibrillation in haemodynamically stable patients with structurally normal hearts should be considered. Cardioversion may be required if the patient remains unstable after prior anticoagulation.[4]

Peripartum cardiomyopathy is an idiopathic cardiomyopathy characterized by heart failure secondary to left ventricular dysfunction. It occurs in late pregnancy and up to 6 months postpartum. Risk factors include multiparity, hypertension, pre-eclampsia, teenage and advanced maternal age, diabetes, family history, ethnicity (African), smoking and prolonged use of β-agonists. Management is as for acute and subsequently chronic heart failure. In haemodynamically stable patients vaginal delivery is preferable, with urgent caesarean delivery being reserved for advanced failure and instability despite treatment, irrespective of gestation. Mortality ranges from 0% to 15%, 50% have persistent deterioration in ventricular function, and there is a 30–50% recurrence risk.

Acute coronary syndromes are rare in pregnancy (0.6–1/10,000 pregnancies) and carry a 5–37% maternal mortality rate. Diagnostic criteria consist of chest pain, electrocardiograph changes and an increase in troponin I level. Risk factors include smoking, hypertension, diabetes, dyslipidaemia, family history, thrombophilia and older age. Beta-blockers and low-dose acetylsalicylic acid (aspirin) are safe, while percutaneous coronary intervention with bare-metal stenting following on from coronary angiogram (with abdominal shielding, brachial or radial access and reduced fluoroscopy time) is preferred to thrombolysis.[5] If possible, delivery should be postponed for at least 2 weeks after infarction, with vaginal delivery usually preferable.[6]

Key summary points

- Management of pregnant women with cardiac disease must be by a multidisciplinary team of obstetrician, cardiologist, obstetric anaesthetist, specialist midwife and haematologist.
- Women with known cardiac disease should have pre-conception assessment and counselling.
- Most patients would be suitable for vaginal delivery, with caesarean section reserved for obstetric reasons.
- Patients with mechanical heart valves have significant risk of thromboembolism.

References

1. Cantwell R, Clutton-Brock T, Cooper G, *et al.* Saving Mothers' Lives: reviewing maternal deaths to make motherhood safer: 2006–2008. The Eighth Report of the Confidential Enquiries into Maternal Deaths in the United Kingdom. *BJOG* 2011; 118 (Supplement 1): 1–203.

2. Royal College of Obstetricians and Gynaecologists. *Cardiac Disease and Pregnancy*. Good Practice No. 13. London: RCOG, 2011.

3. European Society of Cardiology (ESC) Committee for Practice Guidelines. ESC Guidelines on the management of cardiovascular diseases during pregnancy: the Task Force on the Management of Cardiovascular Diseases during Pregnancy of the European Society of Cardiology (ESC). *Eur Heart J* 2011; 32: 3147–97.

4. Adamson DL, Nielson-Percy C. Managing palpitations and arrhythmias during pregnancy. *Heart* 2007; 93: 1630–6.

5. Regitz-Zagrosek V, Seeland U, Geibel-Zehender A, Gohlke-Bärwolf C, Kruck I, Schaefer C. Cardiovascular diseases in pregnancy. *Dtsch Arztebl Int* 2011; 108 (16): 267–73.

6. Kealey AJ. Coronary artery disease and myocardial infarction in pregnancy: a review of epidemiology, diagnosis, and medical and surgical management. *Can J Cardiol* 2010; 26 (6): e185–e189.

9 Alloimmunization in pregnancy

Sarah Vause

Introduction

Alloimmunization is a pathological process, where antibodies are produced against antigens from another individual of the same species. In pregnancy, the mother produces antibodies in response to antigens from the fetus. The most common form of alloimmunization in pregnancy is to the rhesus system of antigens, but other red cell antigens or platelet antigens can also alloimmunize. The antigens are glycoproteins and glycolipids contained within the cell membrane. They vary between individuals (polymorphisms) and the immune system recognizes them as 'self' or 'non-self'.

During pregnancy, blood cells from the fetus may cross the placenta into the maternal circulation. If the fetal antigens are different from the maternal antigens (e.g. RhD-positive fetus in RhD-negative mother) this stimulates an immune response in the mother and production of antibodies. Maternal antibodies (IgG) to the blood cell can then freely cross the placenta into the fetal circulation and bind with the relevant antigen on the fetal blood cell, which is then destroyed. With antibodies to red blood cell antigens, this results in haemolysis and fetal anaemia. With antiplatelet antibodies it results in fetal thrombocytopenia, putting the fetus at risk of intracerebral haemorrhage.

In subsequent pregnancies the antibody response is greater, resulting in more severe disease. Red cell alloimmunization is more likely to occur if the mother and fetus are ABO compatible (ABO incompatible cells in the maternal circulation are destroyed more quickly, before there is time to stimulate an immune response).

Fetal alloimmune disease can be predicted, prevented and treated. This chapter will discuss all three.

Prediction

A blood group and antibody screen should be performed on all women booking for antenatal care. This is a good screening test, as effective intervention is

Antenatal Disorders for the MRCOG and Beyond, Second Edition, ed. Dilly Anumba and Shehnaaz Jivraj.
Published by Cambridge University Press. © Cambridge University Press 2016.

available, either to prevent rhesus alloimmunization occurring if the antibody screen is negative, or to monitor and treat the fetus if the antibody screen is positive.

National Institute for Health and Care Excellence (NICE) guidelines recommend that all women should be offered a further antibody screen at 28 weeks gestation (not just RhD-negative women).[1]

At present screening for platelet alloimmunization is not offered in the UK.

Prevention

RhD alloimmunization can be effectively prevented by the administration of anti-D immunoglobulin to the mother. At present RhD is the only form of alloimmunization for which prevention is available.

Sensitization can occur following recognized potentially sensitizing events (Table 9.1), or following 'silent' fetomaternal haemorrhage. Silent fetomaternal haemorrhage is most common in the third trimester of pregnancy. Following the successful implementation of anti-D prophylaxis in response to potentially sensitizing events (Table 9.2), including delivery (Table 9.3), silent fetomaternal

---

Table 9.1   Potentially sensitizing events

Vaginal bleeding. It is not necessary to administer anti-D for threatened or complete miscarriages < 12 weeks.

Give anti-D to all women having medical or surgical evacuation of uterus, termination of pregnancy (medical or surgical) and all women with ectopic pregnancy, regardless of whether it is treated medically or surgically.

Invasive procedures such as chorionic villus sampling (CVS), amniocentesis

External cephalic version

Falls, trauma, domestic violence – anti-D prophylaxis can be forgotten in the absence of overt bleeding

Delivery

Table 9.2   Dose of anti-D in response to potentially sensitizing events in pregnancy

250 iu before 20 weeks

500 iu and a Kleihauer at or after 20 weeks 0 days

500 iu of anti-D will usually cover a 4 mL fetomaternal bleed

A test for fetomaternal haemorrhage will quantify the requirement for more anti-D

Anti-D should be given within 72 hours of a potentially sensitizing event. However, some protection is obtained if it is administered up to 10 days after the event.

A Kleihauer is an acid elution test which quantifies number of fetal cells in maternal circulation. Flow cytometry can also be used and has advantages in certain situations.

Anti-D should be given intramuscularly into the deltoid muscle

Table 9.3 Care after delivery (UK guidelines – other countries may be different)

Cord blood to check blood group of baby, direct Coombs test and Kleihauer

Kleihauer test should be done within 2 hours of delivery

If baby is RhD negative – do nothing, as will not cause sensitization

If RhD positive – give 500 iu and await Kleihauer to see if more is needed. A dose of 500 iu of anti-D will neutralize up to 4 ml of fetomaternal haemorrhage. Only 1% of women will have a fetomaternal haemorrhage of > 4 ml at delivery, and therefore need more anti-D.

If a woman is already known to be sensitized she does not require anti-D – the aim of giving anti-D is to prevent sensitization.

haemorrhage now accounts for the greatest proportion of new sensitizations. For this reason a programme of routine antenatal anti-D prophylaxis has been introduced.

SILENT SENSITIZATION

Approximately 1.5% of RhD-negative women are sensitized each year (1000 women per year in the UK). Most of these (55–80%) are now due to asymptomatic fetomaternal bleeds known as silent sensitization (although some may be due to failure to administer anti-D in response to recognized potentially sensitizing events). Sensitization due to asymptomatic fetomaternal bleeding is rare before 28 weeks, but increases towards term.

In 2009 NICE guidelines recommended routine antenatal anti-D prophylaxis (RAADP) to all non-sensitized RhD-negative pregnant women in the third trimester.[2] It was estimated that this would reduce the rate of sensitization from 1.5% to 0.2%. Different regimes are used, depending on the way in which services are organized locally. Either one dose of 1500 iu anti-D can be given at 28 weeks, or a two-dose regime can be used, with 500 iu anti-D given at 28 and 34 weeks. The one-dose regime may be easier to organize, but there are some concerns that women may not be protected at the end of pregnancy if the pregnancy goes post term.

The RAADP programme to prevent silent sensitization runs alongside the management of potentially sensitizing events. Even if a woman has received RAADP recently, potentially sensitizing events should still be managed as outlined above.

CONSENT AND REFUSAL

Anti-D is a blood product. Women who are eligible for RAADP should receive written information before making an informed decision about opting for treatment. Consent should be obtained and recorded in the case notes.[3]

FETAL GENOTYPING

At present all RhD-negative women are offered RAADP. However, a proportion of these (40%) will not be at risk of silent sensitization as their fetus will be RhD negative, and therefore some women are given anti-D when it is not necessary. Fetal blood group can be determined from cell-free fetal DNA amplified by polymerase chain reaction (cffDNA PCR). If RhD-positive DNA is found in a pregnant RhD-negative woman, then that DNA must have come from the fetus, and the fetus must be RhD positive. By genotyping the fetus, RAADP could be targeted at those women known to have an RhD-positive fetus. Although this is not current practice, it is likely that a Health Technology Assessment will be carried out to inform NICE guidance and clinical practice in the future.

Treatment

RED BLOOD CELL ALLOIMMUNIZATION

If there is a positive antibody screen for any of the blood group antibodies associated with alloimmune haemolytic disease, then further testing should occur to quantify/titrate the antibody level. Results should be clearly documented in the notes. The woman should be informed of the results and the implications, and a full history taken (Table 9.4).

INVESTIGATION

The history then helps to put further investigation results into context. Repeat quantifications/titrations of antibody levels can be compared with those in previous pregnancies, and give a general impression of risk. Some women have more aggressive antibodies than others, and in one woman the fetus may be more severely affected than in another woman with the same quantification, so it is important to interpret the antibody quantification in the light of the past history. The rate of rise of antibodies may be predictive of worsening disease.

Table 9.4 Issues to be covered in taking a history from a woman with a positive antibody screen
Doses of prophylactic anti-D in this pregnancy
Any previously affected fetus/baby
How serious was it?
• Quantification/titres in previous pregnancy
• Intervention during pregnancy – in-utero transfusion
• Intervention postnatally – phototherapy, top-up transfusion, exchange transfusion
Paternal genotype – may have been checked previously
Paternity – has there been a change of partner since the previous pregnancy

Paternal blood group and genotype can be checked to estimate whether the fetus is at risk, but this assumes that paternity is accurately attributed. A more accurate way of assessing fetal risk (and ascertaining the fetal blood group) is to send maternal blood for testing for cffDNA.

Previously amniocentesis would have been performed to assess the degree of haemolysis by measuring the change in the optical density (OD 450). This reflected the yellowness of the amniotic fluid due to the presence of bilirubin and was used to guide the timing of intrauterine transfusion, by plotting the measurement on Whitfield or Liley charts. Amniocentesis could potentiate the disease by causing further sensitization and a rise in antibody level and is now largely outdated, being replaced by non-invasive methods.

Kell antibodies deserve a special mention, as they behave slightly differently by also causing suppression of haemopoiesis in the fetus. Therefore the antibody quantification for Kell antibodies does not relate as well to degree of anaemia in the fetus, and the OD 450 at amniocentesis is less predictive, as anaemia is not necessarily due to haemolysis.

ULTRASOUND MONITORING

The management of alloimmunized pregnancies has been revolutionized by Doppler ultrasound monitoring of middle cerebral artery (MCA) peak systolic velocity. If a fetus is anaemic the blood flows faster in its circulation, and the peak systolic velocity of blood flow in the MCA can be measured using ultrasound.

This requires technical care, measuring close to the origin of the vessel from the circle of Willis and correcting appropriately for the angle of insonation to estimate the velocity accurately (Figure 9.1). Measurements can be performed from 18 weeks gestation as frequently as required (weekly or 2-weekly is usually appropriate). The measured velocity is then plotted against a reference chart at the appropriate gestation, to determine how likely it is that the fetus is severely anaemic and in need of transfusion.

Following transfusion, the MCA peak systolic velocity measurements can again be used to assess the degree of anaemia and plan subsequent transfusions. MCA peak systolic velocity measurements are useful for all causes of anaemia, including Kell alloimmunization and anaemia due to non-alloimmune causes, e.g. parvovirus.

Late signs which may be seen on ultrasound suggestive of established severe disease include increased liquor volume, scalp oedema, ascites, pleural effusions and a pericardial effusion.

CORDOCENTESIS AND INTRAUTERINE TRANSFUSION

If the fetus is suspected to be severely anaemic, then the treatment options are intrauterine transfusion or delivery and neonatal treatment (phototherapy,

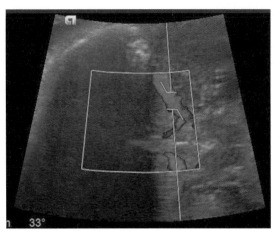

Figure 9.1 Measurement of middle cerebral artery peak systolic velocity. This is an ultrasound image of the fetal head, taken in transverse section at the level of the base of the skull. Colour Doppler has been used to visualize the circle of Willis, and the two middle cerebral arteries (MCAs) can be seen. The Doppler gate has been placed close to the origin of the MCA from the circle of Willis, and an angle correction has been applied to ensure a true reading of the velocity of blood flow. A black and white version of this figure will appear in some formats. For the colour version, please refer to the plate section.

transfusion or exchange transfusion). The choice will depend mainly on the gestation of the pregnancy and to some extent the ease or difficulty of in-utero transfusion in that particular woman.

Intrauterine transfusion should only be performed in tertiary fetal medicine centres. Prior to the transfusion, prophylactic steroids may be given to promote fetal lung maturity, if the pregnancy is at an appropriate gestation. Blood is specially prepared for in-utero transfusion. It is CMV-negative, leucodepleted, irradiated and highly concentrated to reduce the volume which needs to be transfused into the fetal circulation.

Initially, cordocentesis enables accurate determination of fetal haemoglobin. It is usually performed at a point where the cord is static, ideally the placental cord insertion. Sometimes this is not possible because of placental location and fetal lie, and then the fetal umbilical cord insertion can be used, with injection of neuro-muscular blocking drugs to the fetus to temporarily stop fetal movement if necessary.

Once the initial sample has been taken the cordocentesis needle is left in position in the cord, and the donor blood is transfused. The amount of blood required depends on the result of the haemoglobin/haematocrit of the fetus, the haematocrit of the donor unit and the gestation of the pregnancy. There is obviously a larger fetoplacental blood volume at later gestations, and larger volumes of donated blood are needed.

Following transfusion, the needle is flushed with saline and a further sample is taken to assess the post-procedure haemoglobin and haematocrit. The aim is to get the post-transfusion fetal haematocrit to 45%.

The timing of subsequent transfusions can be judged by monitoring fetal MCA Dopplers. Usually there is a need to transfuse approximately 2 weeks later, and transfusions are often continued up to 34 weeks, when delivery of the fetus can be considered.

Potential complications which can be encountered include:

- technical difficulties – especially posterior placenta or obese woman
- cord haematoma
- haemorrhage
- bradycardia
- 1% fetal loss
- preterm delivery

PLANNING FOR DELIVERY

As neonatologists now have less experience with exchange transfusions, owing to the success of antenatal prevention and treatment of alloimmune disease, it seems appropriate to deliver affected babies in a tertiary centre. Delivery should be planned in conjunction with the neonatologists, prophylactic steroids given and appropriate blood available should the baby require exchange transfusion. At delivery, the midwife should be prompted to take cord blood for haemoglobin, Coombs test, blood group and bilirubin level.

If the fetus is affected by RhD alloimmunization the woman will not need any further anti-D – she is already sensitized and has lots of anti-D in her circulation! However, if the fetus is affected by another form of alloimmunization, e.g. Kell, it is important not to overlook anti-D prophylaxis if needed.

Platelet alloimmunization

Platelet alloimmunization is usually only detected after a poor outcome in a previous pregnancy, for example a previous fetus or baby with an intracranial bleed. The platelet antibodies may have been detected as part of the investigations for this (usually HPA-1a or HPA-5b).

As with red cell alloimmunization, assessment of paternal genotype facilitates estimation of the risk to the fetus. Although fetal genotyping is not possible from cffDNA PCR at present, it may be in the future. At present fetal genotype can be determined by chorionic villus sampling or amniocentesis.

Maternal platelet antibody titres do not correlate well with the severity of the disease or the risk to the fetus.

Intravenous immunoglobulin given intravenously weekly to the mother has been shown to improve fetal outcome in some studies. This is an intensive and expensive treatment. Cordocentesis may then be used to determine the fetal platelet count, at which time platelets can be transfused. This raises the fetal platelet count temporarily, but needs to be repeated at frequent intervals, and does not necessarily prevent fetal complications occurring. There are also increased risks associated with the cordocentesis because of the low fetal platelet count, such as increased risk of bleeding or cord haematoma.

If it is anticipated that the fetal platelet count will be low, careful consideration should be given to mode and timing of delivery, in liaison with the neonatal unit. At delivery, cord blood should be taken to check the platelet count of the baby.

It is important to ensure that anti-D is given appropriately to a non-sensitized RhD-negative woman following any invasive procedures to treat platelet alloimmunization (or red cell immunization not due to the D antigen), or delivery.

Key summary points

- Appropriate management of potentially sensitizing events is important to prevent RhD sensitization. Anti-D prophylaxis is often forgotten when women have falls or suffer domestic violence, particularly when there is no overt bleeding.

- Silent fetomaternal haemorrhage now accounts for the greatest proportion of new RhD sensitizations and a large proportion of cases can be prevented by routine antenatal anti-D prophylaxis (RAADP).

- Fetal blood group can be ascertained by testing maternal blood for cell-free fetal DNA (cffDNA).

- Fetal anaemia from any cause can be assessed by measuring the peak systolic velocity of blood flow in the fetal middle cerebral artery. This is particularly useful for Kell alloimmunization.

- If the woman already has RhD antibodies (RhD sensitized) she will not need further anti-D following potentially sensitizing events. If she is sensitized by other antigens, it is important not to overlook anti-D prophylaxis if it is needed.

References

1. National Institute for Health and Care Excellence (NICE); National Collaborating Centre for Women's and Children's Health. *Antenatal Care: Routine Care for the Healthy Pregnant Woman.* NICE Clinical Guideline CG62. London: NICE, 2008.

2. National Institute for Health and Care Excellence (NICE). *Routine Antenatal Anti-D Prophylaxis for Women who are Rhesus D Negative.* NICE Technology Appraisal Guidance TA156. London: NICE, 2008.

3. Royal College of Obstetricians and Gynaecologists. *The Use of Anti-D Immunoglobulin for Rhesus D Prophylaxis.* Green-top Guideline No. 22. London: RCOG, 2011.

Further reading

Mari G, Deter RL, Carpenter RL, *et al.* Noninvasive diagnosis by Doppler ultrasonography of fetal anemia due to maternal red-cell alloimmunization. Collaborative Group for Doppler Assessment of the Blood Velocity in Anemic Fetuses. *N Engl J Med* 2000; 342: 9–14.

10 Maternal mental health disorders

Nusrat Mir and Meena Srinivas

Introduction

Psychiatric disorders during pregnancy and the postnatal period are common and important. They cause significant psychological suffering at a special time in a woman's life, unnecessary maternal misery, impaired maternal bonding and child development, strained relationships, as well as increased risk of obstetric complications.

If not recognized and managed appropriately, their impact can be devastating in the form of suicide and infanticide. The former is recognized as one of the leading indirect causes of maternal death in the UK.[1]

It is therefore vital that an obstetrician is familiar with common perinatal psychiatric disorders and has a basic understanding of their management.[2,3] This chapter focuses on the epidemiology and clinical features of common perinatal psychiatric disorders, offering practical advice on their management.

Psychiatric disorders in pregnancy

DEPRESSION IN PREGNANCY

Incidence

Estimated rates vary from 7–15% in developed countries to 19–25% in underdeveloped countries.

Onset

In women with no past history, new-onset depression peaks during the third trimester. In women with a pre-existing history of depression, recurrence of depression in the first trimester occurs in 50% of cases. This is commonly associated with discontinuation of antidepressant medication around the time of conception.

Antenatal Disorders for the MRCOG and Beyond, Second Edition, ed. Dilly Anumba and Shehnaaz Jivraj. Published by Cambridge University Press. © Cambridge University Press 2016.

Risk factors

- past history of depression
- lack of partner
- relationship difficulties
- young age
- poverty
- poor social support
- unplanned pregnancy

Clinical features

Symptoms and signs of depression during pregnancy do not differ from depression at other times in a woman's life. The only difference is that the content and focus of the depressed woman's negativity is the pregnancy and everything associated with it.

Low mood with tearfulness will be apparent. The woman may notice that she is more prone to mood swings and more emotionally sensitive, which is often blamed on hormonal changes. Motivation can drop, and there is little interest in planning for the baby's arrival. On the contrary, a woman who has previously planned the pregnancy may become ambivalent or negative towards it. In extreme cases, there can be a preoccupation with wanting a termination of pregnancy. Depressed pregnant women may worry excessively about something going seriously wrong with the pregnancy such as a miscarriage, stillbirth or giving birth to a baby with a congenital birth defect. They may become petrified of not being able to get through labour. Severe depression leads to ideas and acts of self-harm or suicide.

Treatment

Good obstetric practice includes being aware of the risk factors for antenatal depression and screening for depressive symptoms at every opportunity, from the first antenatal (booking) appointment to the follow-up appointments in hospital and the community.

The treatment of depression in pregnancy depends on its severity. In cases of mild antenatal depression, psychological interventions such as counselling and cognitive behavioural therapy (CBT) are the main strategy. Moderate depression is unlikely to respond solely to psychological approaches, and antidepressant therapy will need to be considered.

Any decision to prescribe antidepressant medication needs to be made together with the patient after careful weighing up of the risks of the antidepressant and its potential benefits versus the risks of untreated depression in pregnancy (Table 10.1).

Severe depression warrants a combination of antidepressant plus CBT and referral to a specialist perinatal psychiatry service if one exists locally. Where risk

Table 10.1   Risk–benefit analysis

Risk of drugs	Risk of illness
Teratogenicity	Unstable mental state/risk
Neonatal withdrawal syndrome	Stress on fetus
Cognitive/neurobehavioural problems	Poor obstetric outcome
Breastfeeding risks	Low birth weight
	Intrauterine growth restriction
	Poor mother–infant bonding

of suicide or harm to the pregnancy becomes an issue, hospitalization may be needed.

PSYCHOSIS IN PREGNANCY

Clinical features

Psychotic symptoms in pregnancy, such as those of schizophrenia and severe bipolar disorder, do not differ from other times in a woman's life.

Hallucinations in any modality can occur. Most commonly these will be auditory, with the woman complaining of 'hearing voices'. She may also see things when nothing is there (visual hallucinations) or feel things on her skin (tactile hallucinations).

Delusions (fixed false beliefs) that are held with absolute conviction are the other main psychotic symptom, and persecutory delusions are the most common. Other types of delusions that may be evident include grandiose, nihilistic, jealous, hypochondriacal or bizarre.

In chronic schizophrenia, 'negative' symptoms such as affective blunting, poverty of speech (alogia), loss of drive (avolition) and social withdrawal (asociality) may be predominant and disabling.

Bipolar disorder that is unstable presents with hypomania/mania or depression. Hypomania/mania is characterized by elevated mood, overactivity, racing thoughts, grandiose thinking, pressured speech, disinhibition and decreased need for sleep. Depressive symptoms include pervasive low mood, loss of interest and enjoyment (anhedonia), poor concentration, sleep disturbance, negative thinking and hopelessness.

Treatment

Management of pregnant women with psychosis is complex and requires an integrated multidisciplinary approach including psychiatry, obstetrics, paediatrics and social services. The aim is to maximize the mental and physical health of the mother while minimizing any risks to the child. Success hinges on forward planning, joint working and good communication between disciplines.

As a general guide, women with psychosis who become pregnant while on antipsychotic medication will, in the majority of cases, need to continue on it as maintenance therapy. However, it is advisable that the lowest effective dose be used in pregnancy. Abrupt discontinuation of antipsychotic and mood-stabilizing medication (e.g. lithium) should be avoided without discussion with a psychiatrist. Polypharmacy is also best avoided in pregnancy.

As with antidepressant prescribing, any decision to start a new antipsychotic in pregnancy should be made after a full discussion of the risks and benefits of the medication with the pregnant woman. A multidisciplinary pre-birth planning meeting around 30 weeks of gestation is essential in all cases of psychosis and for women at particularly high risk of postpartum psychosis (e.g. women with bipolar disorder).

A prophylactic management plan for prevention of postpartum psychosis needs to be made for all bipolar women, even in cases where the condition has been stable for many years. A recommended strategy is to start such women on a low-dose atypical antipsychotic (e.g. olanzapine) immediately after delivery, and to continue this for at least 3 months into the postnatal period.

General principles of prescribing psychotropic medication in pregnancy are summarized in Table 10.2. Current evidence on the safety profile of psychotropic medication in pregnancy is summarized in Table 10.3.

Postnatal psychiatric disorders

POSTPARTUM BLUES

Incidence
Affects 50–80% of women.

Onset
Typically starts on second or third postnatal day.

Table 10.2	Principles of prescribing psychotropic medication in pregnancy
Careful risk–benefit assessment	
If mild to moderate severity, use non-pharmacological intervention	
Avoid first-trimester exposure if possible	
Choose drugs with lower risk profiles for mother/fetus/infant	
Start at the lowest effective dose and increase slowly	
Avoid abrupt discontinuation of maintenance mood-stabilizing/antipsychotic medication without discussion with psychiatrist	
Avoid polypharmacy if possible	

Table 10.3 Safety profile of psychotropic medication in pregnancy: current evidence

Medication	Evidence
Antidepressants	
Selective serotonin reuptake inhibitors (SSRIs)	
• Fluoxetine	Can be used in pregnancy. Relative risk of birth defects increased but absolute risk small
• Sertraline	
• Citalopram	
• Paroxetine	Not advised in pregnancy
Tricyclic antidepressants (TCAs)	
• Amitriptyline, imipramine, nortriptyline	No convincing data to suggest teratogenicity
Antipsychotics	
Atypical	
• Olanzapine, quetiapine, risperidone	No convincing data to suggest teratogenicity. To be used with caution after discussion with psychiatrists
Typical	
• Trifluperidol, haloperidol	
Mood stabilizers	
• Lithium	Fetal cardiac defects
• Sodium valproate	Fetal neural tube defects
	Both to be avoided if possible

Clinical features

- depressed mood
- tearfulness
- irritability
- emotional lability
- feeling overwhelmed

Prognosis

Transient, self-limiting. Symptoms should start to remit by second week. However, women who experience severe postpartum blues may be up to three times more likely to develop postnatal depression, according to research.

Treatment

No specific treatment other than reassurance and support is required.

POSTNATAL DEPRESSION

Incidence

Affects 10–15% of women at any time in the first 6 months following childbirth.

Onset

May have a gradual or sudden onset and is usually apparent within 2 months of childbirth.

Risk factors

- depression or anxiety during pregnancy
- past history of depression
- past history of other psychiatric illness
- recent stressful life events
- poor social support

Clinical features

A depressed mother may be noticeably weepy and not her normal self. There may be excessive anxiety about the baby's health that cannot be allayed by reassurance. This may lead to sleepless nights in order to watch over the baby and repeated checking behaviour. It may also lead to a preoccupation with the idea that the baby is deformed or physically ill despite evidence to the contrary.

Self-blame can sometimes be evident. A mother may believe that she cannot live up to her own expectations of a 'good mother', and that she is not as competent as her own mother. She may also compare herself unfavourably with others in her peer group, and even remain at home to avoid their criticism. Suicidal thoughts or fear of harming the baby, irritability and loss of libido affect some women with more severe depression. The last of these can lead to significant relationship conflict in a previously harmonious couple (Table 10.4).

Treatment

The treatment of postnatal depression depends on a variety of factors. These include the severity of depression, presence of psychiatric comorbidity (e.g. alcohol

Table 10.4   Clinical features of postnatal depression
Persistent low mood and tearfulness
Loss of interest and enjoyment
Sleep disturbance
Low confidence/self-esteem ('bad mother')
Difficulty coping with childcare
Difficulty bonding
Extreme anxiety about health of baby
Over-concern about baby's feeding/sleeping regime
Physical anxiety symptoms/panic attacks
Suicidal thoughts
Infanticidal thoughts
Relationship difficulties/conflict

misuse, personality disorder), level of risk of suicide or harm to the baby, and presence of social support.

The National Institute for Health and Care Excellence (NICE) guidelines on antenatal and postnatal mental health indicate that optimal treatment is based on a stepped-care model in which mild to moderate illness is treated in primary care, moderate to severe illness may need input from secondary care, and severe, complex illness is the realm of secondary care or a specialist perinatal mental health service if one exists locally.[3]

The first-line treatment of mild postnatal depression is non-directive counselling, support and understanding. Moderate postnatal depression is unlikely to respond to counselling alone. Moreover, formal psychological intervention such as CBT and/or antidepressant therapy may be required.

Breastfeeding is not a contraindication to antidepressant therapy. However, in breastfeeding women, the risk–benefit balance of antidepressant drugs is altered, with a consequent shift in emphasis towards psychological therapies. If an antidepressant is considered, the choice will depend on the patient's preference, previous response to treatment, local availability of psychological therapies, the severity of the illness and the risks involved.[4]

Certain antidepressants are considered safer than others in breastfeeding women, but in general the long-term outcomes for exposed babies are unknown. Sertraline and imipramine are preferred antidepressants, as they pass into breast-milk at relatively low levels.

If the depression is severe, complicated by suicidal or infanticidal ideas or child protection issues, a referral to secondary care or a specialist perinatal mental health service is indicated. Cases of recurrent depression or those with comorbidity, such as alcohol misuse or personality disorder, should be referred. In some cases, severe postnatal depression will require inpatient treatment in a specialist mother and baby unit, with or without use of the Mental Health Act.

POSTPARTUM (PUERPERAL) PSYCHOSIS

Incidence
1–2 cases per 1000 deliveries. Women with bipolar disorder have a significantly increased risk; they have a 1 in 4 chance of suffering from postpartum psychosis.

Onset
The onset is sudden, most commonly occurring within 2–4 weeks of delivery.

Risk factors
- past history of postpartum psychosis
- family history of postpartum psychosis
- past history of bipolar disorder

Clinical features

The early signs of postpartum psychosis are often non-specific, for example insomnia, agitation, perplexity and odd behaviour. Such symptoms can be easily overlooked or attributed to postpartum blues, and their significance not recognized. However, the patient may be floridly psychotic within hours, as onset is frequently very rapid. Postpartum psychosis has been described as a 'kaleidoscopic' illness, because the symptoms and signs fluctuate and quickly change from one thing to another.[5]

Mood symptoms are prominent. Typically these may include elation, lability of mood, rambling speech and overactivity. In some cases, the mood is one of depression.

Classic psychotic symptoms such as delusions and hallucinations also occur. The delusions may be of any type including persecutory, grandiose or jealousy. Their content may be bizarre and may involve the baby. They are more likely to be fleeting and less systematized than might be found in acute schizophrenia. Hallucinations are most likely to be in the auditory modality, though visual, olfactory, tactile and gustatory have also been described. In rare cases there may be command auditory hallucinations ordering the mother to harm her baby.

Perplexity and confusion, which may fluctuate from hour to hour, is one of the hallmarks of postpartum psychosis. Mixing in with the sudden mood changes, delusional thinking and hallucinatory experiences, it serves to make postpartum psychosis a most devastating and frightening illness (Table 10.5).

Treatment

Postpartum psychosis is a psychiatric emergency, as it carries risk not only to the mother but also to her baby. Urgent referral to a psychiatrist is therefore essential to enable a full assessment of the mother's mental state and an appropriate treatment plan to be instituted.

In the vast majority of cases, postpartum psychosis requires management in a hospital setting, ideally in a specialized mother and baby unit. If one does not exist locally, efforts should be made to transfer the mother and baby to the nearest regional unit (Table 10.6). Admission may require use of the Mental Health Act

---

Table 10.5 Clinical features of postpartum (puerperal) psychosis

Mood symptoms
- Depressed mood, lability, elation, rambling speech, overactivity

Psychotic symptoms
- Delusions – fleeting not fixed, systematization not usual re baby, mood incongruent, persecutory, reference, jealous, grandiose
- Hallucinations – auditory, visual, olfactory, tactile

Perplexity and confusion

Table 10.6   Who to refer to a specialist perinatal psychiatry service (or general psychiatry service where specialist service is unavailable)

Women with current symptoms of psychosis, severe anxiety or severe depression

Women expressing ideas of self-harm, suicide or homicide

Women with a history of bipolar disorder, schizophrenia or other psychoses

Women with a previous history of postpartum (puerperal) psychosis

Women with a history of serious mental illness on complex psychotropic medication regimes

Women with a history of serious mental illness who are considering pregnancy (pre-conception counselling)

Adapted from: RCOG Good Practice Guide No.14, *Management of Women with Mental Health Issues during Pregnancy and the Postnatal Period.*[2]

(involuntary admission) in severe cases. The alternatives will be admission to an acute general psychiatric ward or intensive community home treatment.

Most women will require antipsychotic medication in addition to antidepressants and/or mood stabilizers, depending on the precise nature of the episode. If agitation is severe, intramuscular antipsychotic medication may be necessary. Care should, however, be taken not to over-sedate a woman caring for an infant, particularly if she is breastfeeding and needs to do night feeds. In cases where severe depressive features with psychomotor retardation are present, electroconvulsive therapy (ECT) may be indicated.

Conclusion

Pregnancy and childbirth can exacerbate pre-existing mental disorders or precipitate new episodes of depression, anxiety and psychosis. Optimal obstetric care means screening for past and present mental health problems at the booking clinic, early identification of high-risk patients, and referral to a specialist perinatal psychiatry service or general adult psychiatry team if no specialist service exists locally.

Good communication and joint working between obstetric and psychiatric services, with clear management plans, is the key to improving a woman's quality of life in the perinatal period and preventing unnecessary perinatal psychiatric morbidity and mortality.

Key summary points

- Perinatal psychiatric disorders are one of the leading indirect causes of maternal mortality.
- Pregnancy and childbirth can exacerbate pre-existing psychiatric disorders or trigger new episodes of depression, anxiety and psychosis, whose impact on mother and child can be devastating.

- Risk–benefit analysis involves assessing the potential effect of psychiatric illness on the mother, fetus and family, and potential effects of psychotropic treatment on the mother and fetus.

- Postpartum psychosis has a sudden onset and rapid progression, making it a psychiatric emergency.

- Successful management of women with perinatal psychiatric disorders is based on early screening and referral, effective multidisciplinary joint working and forward planning.

References

1. Cantwell R, Clutton-Brock T, Cooper G, *et al.* Saving Mothers' Lives: reviewing maternal deaths to make motherhood safer: 2006–2008. The Eighth Report of the Confidential Enquiries into Maternal Deaths in the United Kingdom. *BJOG* 2011; 118 (Supplement 1): 1–203.

2. Royal College of Obstetricians and Gynaecologists. *Management of Women with Mental Health Issues during Pregnancy and the Postnatal Period.* Good Practice Guide No. 14. London: RCOG, 2011.

3. National Institute for Health and Care Excellence (NICE). *Antenatal and Postnatal Mental Health: Clinical Management and Service Guidance.* NICE Clinical Guideline CG45. London: NICE, 2007.

4. Mir N. Postnatal depression: when is medication the answer? *Women's Health Journal* (Primary Care) 2012; 14 (1): 31–4.

5. Sit D, Rothschild AJ, Wisner KL. A review of postpartum psychosis. *J Womens Health* 2006; 15: 352–68.

Further reading

Henshaw C, Cox J, Barton J. *Modern Management of Perinatal Psychiatric Disorders.* London: Royal College of Psychiatrists, 2009.

Lanza di Scalea T, Wisner K. Antidepressant use during breastfeeding. *Clin Obstet Gynecol* 2009; 52: 483–97.

O'Keane V, Marsh M, Seneviratne G. *Psychiatric disorders and Pregnancy.* London: Taylor & Francis, 2006.

11 Drug and alcohol misuse in pregnancy

Julia Bodle

Introduction

The 2006–08 Centre for Maternal and Child Enquiries (CMACE) report highlighted 35 maternal deaths related to substance misuse in the UK.[1] By comparison, 53 women died from cardiac disease and 36 from neurological conditions, making substance misusers an important subgroup of women who died during or within 1 year of childbirth. This was the third CMACE report to draw attention to this area of maternal health, but what such a report cannot, by its nature, assess is the significant maternal morbidity underpinning the mortality rates in this group, nor the effects of substance misuse on partners and children. It is estimated that between 250,000 and 350,000 children in the UK are living with one or more parents who misuse substances.

Pregnancy is often the trigger to wider health and social interventions, presenting a unique opportunity for professionals to engage with women and their families and provide support, which can facilitate lifelong change. Good outcomes require a true multidisciplinary and inter-agency approach involving primary, secondary and tertiary care; NHS, social care, private and voluntary sectors, with robust pathways for sharing information.

In this chapter, substance misuse and how it affects the pregnant woman and her unborn child is discussed. An outline is provided of how maternity services can intervene to improve maternal and fetal health, as well as the health of her partner and her existing children.

What is substance misuse?

The consumption of mood-altering substances is the natural state of humankind throughout its existence, with each society adopting its own accepted drugs. Caffeine, alcohol and nicotine are acceptable and legal in many modern societies. However, legality does not equate to safety. Cocaine was a constituent of the drink

Antenatal Disorders for the MRCOG and Beyond, Second Edition, ed. Dilly Anumba and Shehnaaz Jivraj. Published by Cambridge University Press. © Cambridge University Press 2016.

Coca Cola until 1903. Morphine was widely available without prescription in the UK until 1920. Cannabis was legally available in the UK until 1928, and amphetamines were widely available over the counter in pharmacies as 'pep pills' until the 1950s. Furthermore, there are numerous 'legal highs' available today.

ACCEPTED DEFINITIONS OF SUBSTANCE MISUSE

Problem drug use is any drug use which has serious negative consequences of a physical, psychological, social, interpersonal, financial or legal nature for the user and those around them. This is usually heavy use with features of dependence.

Substance misuse is an illness where choice has been removed by the effects on cognitive function of the substance(s) taken. It should be viewed as a chronic relapsing and remitting illness, whose damaging effects need to be managed through harm reduction and stabilization. This is the mainstay of the management of substance misuse in pregnancy.

Problem alcohol use is hazardous drinking with regular consumption of 3 units or more of alcohol per day, or more than 14 units per week for women. This also includes binge drinking: consumption of more than 6 units of alcohol on any one occasion even if weekly limits are not exceeded. The term *harmful drinking* is employed when there is a pattern of drinking that causes damage to the physical or mental health of the user or others (ICD-10 criteria[2]).

Drug and alcohol dependence includes a cluster of behavioural, cognitive and physiological phenomena that develop after repeated substance use (ICD-10 criteria[2]). The features of such dependence include:

- a strong desire to take the substance
- a higher priority given to substance use than to other activities and obligations
- difficulties controlling use
- persisting in use despite harmful consequences
- increased tolerance to a substance
- a physical withdrawal state

How common is substance misuse in pregnancy?

Quantifying the prevalence of alcohol and drug misuse during pregnancy is difficult; pregnant women do not tend to voluntarily disclose their substance misuse and/or the extent of it. Government statistics suggest that 30% of women of reproductive age consume alcohol above recommended levels (14 units per week), and 16% of all women are thought to have levels of alcohol consumption which are hazardous. Approximately 9% of the adult population of England and Wales have used illicit drugs in the preceding year, with 3% reporting using a class A drug. Cannabis is the commonest drug of misuse, followed by cocaine.

Substances of misuse

Table 11.1 is not a comprehensive list of substances of misuse, but includes those commonly brought to the attention of healthcare professionals. Other illicit drugs not listed include lysergic acid diethylamide (LSD) and 'magic mushrooms'. Prescribed drugs of misuse include quetiapine, mirtazapine, risperidone, pregabalin, gabapentin, carbamazepine and many others.

Table 11.1 Substances of misuse

Drug	Usual form	Effects	Route of administration
Alcohol Legal	Liquid	Central nervous system depressant Disinhibition may lead to aggression or risk-taking behaviour, toxicity, loss of consciousness and death Long-term liver, brain, heart, stomach damage and obesity	Oral liquid
Cannabis Class B[*]	Resin Buds Synthetic Oil	Relaxant, mild intoxicant Sleepiness and heightened sensations Long-term apathy, poor memory and rarely psychosis	Usually smoked with tobacco, can be eaten
Heroin Class A[*]	Brown powder	Opiate Intoxication followed by drowsiness, cardiac and respiratory depression Long-term addiction, intense craving and withdrawal.	Smoked Injected
Methadone Class A[*]	Green liquid Tablets	Opiate Intoxication	Swallowed
Buprenorphine	Tablets	Opiate partial agonist Intoxication	Snorted Sublingual Can be injected
Codeine Class B[*] Legal (lower doses)	Tablets	Opiate Intoxication	Swallowed
Benzodiazepines Class C[*]	Tablets	Central nervous system depressant	Swallowed Can be injected
Cocaine and crack cocaine Class A[*]	Powder Rocks	CNS stimulant Increases heart rate, respiratory rate, blood pressure, dilates pupils, euphoria, energy and confidence, anxiety, paranoia Long-term depression, lethargy, lack of sleep, eating disorders	Snorted (powder or crushed tablets) Swallowed (tablets or powder) Smoked (crystals) IV (powder)

Table 11.1 (*cont.*)

Drug	Usual form	Effects	Route of administration
Amphetamines, mephedrone Class B*	Powder Tablets Crystals	CNS stimulant Increases heart rate, respiratory rate, blood pressure, dilates pupils, increases feelings of energy and confidence, anxiety, paranoia Long-term depression, lethargy, lack of sleep, eating disorders	Snorted (powder or crushed tablets) Swallowed (tablets or powder) Smoked (crystals) IV (powder)
Ketamine Class C*	Liquid (medical grade) Powder Tablets	Out-of-body experience, hallucinations, muscle weakness, and confusion Long-term bladder problems, cognitive impairment	Snorted (powder) Swallowed (tablets) Injected (liquid)
Ecstasy Class A*	Tablets Powder	Heightened sensations and 'love', sometimes anxiety	Swallowed Smoked or snorted (crushed tablets or powder)
Solvents Legal	Aerosol	Central nervous system depressant with effects similar to alcohol Long-term damage to brain, muscle, liver, kidneys	Inhaled
Cyclizine	Tablets	Potentiates effects of opiates Hallucinogenic at high doses	Swallowed Injected (crushed tablets usually)

*The Misuse of Drugs Act 1971 sets out three categories, class A, class B and class C. Class A drugs are those deemed most dangerous, and carry the harshest punishments. Class C represents those deemed to have the least capacity for harm, which carry more lenient punishment. This classification is contentious because in reality the potential harm has little bearing on the class.

Effects of substances of misuse on pregnancy

Many women who drink alcohol to excess and use illicit drugs also struggle with mental health problems and other comorbid behaviours such as smoking, poor nutrition, complex social factors and poor attendance for antenatal care, which can all contribute to poor pregnancy outcome. It is therefore impossible to evaluate the risks of specific drugs to mother and baby in isolation. However, below is an attempt to do so.

ALCOHOL

Alcohol is teratogenic and fetotoxic with a dose-dependent effect. It can affect the entire reproductive process, the most vulnerable time for the fetus being before

10 weeks gestation. The level and pattern of consumption is important, with binge drinking being more harmful than daily drinking with the same weekly unit consumption. Controversy exists over whether infrequent low levels of alcohol consumption cause harm.

Associated problems
- infertility
- miscarriage
- aneuploidy
- congenital anomaly
- fetal growth restriction (FGR), dose response
- preterm labour
- perinatal death
- neonatal abstinence syndrome (NAS)
- fetal alcohol syndrome (FAS) and fetal alcohol spectrum disorders (FASD)

CANNABIS

Cannabis is usually a mild intoxicant, but 1 in 10 users may experience confusion, hallucinations, anxiety and paranoia. The fat-soluble active ingredients can build up in the brain with regular use, causing apathy, poor concentration, poor short-term memory and sometimes psychosis. Data on the effects in pregnancy are poor and difficult to separate from those caused by tobacco, with which it is usually smoked.

Associated problems
- associated with tobacco use (preterm delivery, FGR, NAS, sudden infant death syndrome)
- mild NAS (36 hours)
- neurodevelopmental disorders
- poor parenting

HEROIN

There are no specific effects of heroin on pregnancy, but its short half-life (6 hours) causes repeated withdrawal, which can lead to miscarriage.

Associated problems
- first-trimester miscarriage
- stillbirth
- preterm delivery
- NAS (24–36 hours)

METHADONE

The long half-life of methadone (72 hours) reduces withdrawal symptoms and delays NAS (36–72 hours).

BUPRENORPHINE

The long half-life of buprenorphine (37 hours) reduces withdrawal symptoms and delays NAS.

CODEINE

Codeine is thought to be safe during pregnancy, although there is little evidence regarding misuse. Its short half-life may predispose to withdrawal and problems similar to heroin as well as NAS (24–36 hours).

BENZODIAZEPINES

There is little conclusive evidence of direct harm to the pregnancy or the fetus, but most studies are on low doses. There is an association with cleft palate.

Associated problems
- cleft palate
- NAS (7–10 days, can be severe and prolonged)
- concerns regarding brain development and FGR

COCAINE/CRACK COCAINE, AMPHETAMINES AND MEPHEDRONE

These stimulant drugs are quickly absorbed, inhibiting dopamine and serotonin reuptake in the brain, causing euphoria. The excess neurotransmitters then cause sympathetic nervous system stimulation: tachycardia, hypertension and vasoconstriction. Pregnancy harm is thought to arise from the consequences of vasoconstriction on the placenta, uterus and fetus.

Associated problems
- miscarriage
- FGR
- stillbirth (4–25%)
- abruption (10–19% with cocaine)
- preterm labour
- urinary tract anomalies
- limb reduction defects
- ischaemic brain abnormalities

- intestinal atresia
- NAS, may last 8–10 weeks
- possible childhood behavioural problems

KETAMINE

Ketamine is a general anaesthetic that produces muscle relaxation and reduced pain sensation. It also stimulates the sympathetic peripheral nervous system, causing tachycardia, hypertension, bronchodilation and diarrhoea. There is little known about its effects on pregnancy, but it may be associated with hypotonia in the newborn.

ECSTASY

Ecstasy is an indirect monoaminergic agonist and serotonin reuptake inhibitor. There is little known about its effects on pregnancy, but it may be associated with delayed motor development in infancy.

SOLVENTS

There is little known about their effects on pregnancy, but they may be associated with preterm delivery and congenital abnormalities.

'LEGAL' HIGHS

These are drugs that produce similar effects to illegal drugs (central nervous system stimulation, depression or hallucination) but are not illegal. There is little information about the medical consequences of taking these drugs. It is likely, however, that those producing stimulant effects may cause problems during pregnancy similar to other stimulant drugs.

General principles of management

PHILOSOPHY OF CARE

The general principles of managing substance misuse across the UK have been summarized in a Department of Health monograph, and the same principles apply during pregnancy.[3] The care philosophy that should pertain especially during pregnancy has also been detailed in several guidance documents produced by the National Collaborating Centre for Women's and Children's Health and the National Institute for Health and Care Excellence (NICE).[4] These are briefly outlined as follows:

- Encourage the woman to attend regularly for antenatal care.
- Encourage the woman and her partner to engage in treatment for their substance misuse.

- Normalize maternity care as much as possible, while recognizing the social and medical problems associated with substance misuse.
- Provide accurate and honest advice regarding the risks of substance misuse to the woman and her baby.
- Ensure that regular communication exists between all professionals, so that advice is consistent, and that any concerns are dealt with appropriately.
- Provide an individualized multi-agency care plan consistent with minimizing harm and stabilizing lifestyle.
- Following birth, promote bonding and facilitate good parenting skills.
- Provide family planning and sexual health advice.

ATTITUDE

There is a prevailing misconception in society that women who misuse substances are less deserving of medical and social care than those who do not, and that they make unfit mothers. This attitude, with its concomitant fear of judgement and having a child removed, can lead to the non-disclosure of substance misuse and is the single most important barrier to effective and safe care for this group of women. It is therefore imperative for healthcare professionals to adopt an attitude which projects an understanding that substance misuse is a chronic disease of a relapsing and remitting nature that is not the 'fault' of the patient. Substance misuse and parenting are not mutually exclusive, and the best place of care for the majority of children is with their mother.

HOLISTIC CARE

Women who misuse substances often have comorbid medical conditions whose management is compromised by their substance misuse. Pregnancy presents an opportunity to address these problems by opportunistic assessment, facilitating referral to specialist services, coordinating and providing transport to appointments to assist with attendance.

Comorbid medical problems
- psychiatric disorders
- dental problems
- superficial abscess from injecting – groin, skin from 'skin popping' (see below)
- liver problems – hepatitis C, alcoholic liver disease
- lung problems from inhaling drugs
- pancreatitis – alcohol
- subacute bacterial endocarditis (SBE)
- poor nutrition and anaemia

- accidental injury when intoxicated
- overdose

Poverty and social deprivation are often associated with substance misuse, which in turn worsens social circumstances. These circumstances often pose the most pressing problems, and help should be offered in parallel with medical care.

Social problems
- lack of family support
- social isolation
- lack of education
- poor finances
- criminal activity
- poor housing
- domestic violence
- prostitution

Women can be helped to access services such as adult education programmes, the benefit agency, housing services and legal services as needed.

Holistic care should include the care of the partner and existing children. Partners who misuse substance should be encouraged to seek help. Smoking cessation advice should be given to both parents. General enquiries about other children should also be made, for example about their motor or speech development or schooling. The aim is not to provide comprehensive services for the whole family through the maternity services, but to be alert to any obvious or serious problems.

ENGAGEMENT

Women do not engage with services for many reasons. They may have poor organizational skills, or they may be trying to conceal their substance misuse or avoiding social services involvement. Whatever the reason, late booking (after 18 weeks) and poor attendance are common in this group and are associated with poor outcomes.

Every contact with maternity services should be used as an opportunity to engage with the mother, her partner and her family in a non-judgemental and supportive way. The focus should be on how maternity care can help achieve a positive outcome for the whole family. The attitude of staff and a holistic approach to care helps to facilitate engagement. For those who do not engage, maternity services must have robust systems for follow-up.

Table 11.2   Roles and responsibilities of those involved in providing maternity care for women affected by substance misuse

Community midwife	Provides routine antenatal care, refers to specialist services
General practitioner	Provides treatment support in between pregnancies and works closely with community midwife
Specialist midwife	Works alongside community midwife and consultant, coordinates care
Obstetrician	Responsible for the care of women with obstetric risk factors
Substance misuse service	Multidisciplinary treatment programme
Anaesthetist	Assessment and management of anaesthetic risk
Infectious diseases midwife	Assists with specialist aspects of care
Paediatrician	Assessment and management of neonatal risk
Health visitor	Liaison with woman's health visitor

COMMUNICATION

Communication is crucial to effective and safe care and requires a central person, the specialist substance misuse midwife, to coordinate care, ensuring communication across the multiple agencies involved. That person can then ensure that all professionals are aware of all aspects of the woman's medical and social care and facilitate the woman's engagement with all aspects of her care.

MODEL OF CARE

This differs with place of practice but is best underpinned by a shared-care multiagency philosophy. Disclosure of substance misuse during pregnancy should trigger a referral to the specialist substance misuse maternity services, who then facilitate referral to all the relevant substance misuse and social care services as appropriate (Table 11.2).

Pre-conception care

As with other chronic conditions, the aim of pre-conception care is to achieve stability through engagement with specialist services in order to optimize health status prior to embarking on a pregnancy, thereby improving the outcome for mother and baby. The barriers to achieving this are the same as those encountered with other chronic conditions. Stable or 'well-controlled' patients attend specialist services, plan their pregnancies and do well; unstable patients do not.

Pre-conception care should be offered to all women of reproductive age who misuse substances by the doctors they regularly see, be they in general practice or specialist services. It should include additional components specific to optimizing pregnancy outcome. Any woman of reproductive age should routinely receive advice, when appropriate, for the following:

- smoking cessation
- fertility control, including contraception and unwanted pregnancy
- cervical smears
- sexually transmitted infections and blood-borne viruses (BBV)
- planned pregnancy, including pre-conception folic acid, vitamin D, healthy diet, smoking cessation, rubella and BBV testing

Antenatal care

Women who do not have obstetric or other risk factors are suitable for antenatal care led by their midwife. Their primary care provider can be the community midwife. The specialist midwife in substance misuse can coordinate and liaise between all the professionals involved in the care of the woman. Women with obstetric risk factors should be seen and assessed by an obstetrician with an interest and expertise in providing such care, who should lead their care.

IDENTIFICATION OF PATIENTS

Enquiry regarding past and present drug and alcohol use should be routinely made for all maternity booking appointments. This should include over-the-counter and prescription drugs, e.g. codeine. Staff should be trained to use standard protocols to assess whether referral to specialist services is needed. Where there is disclosed or suspected ongoing substance misuse, women should be referred. Women with past substance misuse may be referred, depending on local protocols and resources.

Some women conceal their substance misuse; even robust systems may identify only half of those affected. Women sometimes move their care, book late, or book outside their place of residence to conceal substance misuse. These women may be identified though safeguarding processes, postnatally when the baby develops NAS, or not at all. All staff need to have a high index of suspicion in all pregnancies.

MANAGEMENT OF SUBSTANCE MISUSE

Assessment

Drug use

- clarify all drugs used – some women only disclose 'important' drugs and not others, e.g. cannabis, benzodiazepines
- daily drug(s) used, dose or money spent, e.g. £30 heroin daily (street value gives an idea of purity and financial implications)
- method of use – smoked, snorted, swallowed, etc.
- daily pattern – e.g., how many times a day; is some left over for the morning?
- inspect any injection sites for infection or venous damage

Alcohol use

- total weekly units
- pattern of drinking – daily/binge

Both

- length of use
- triggers
- attempts to cut down/stop use
- partner and/or family aware of use
- family/peer support
- does partner/other family member use?
- any agency support – e.g. drug/alcohol services, housing, probation, etc.

Antenatal screening and investigations

- routine antenatal screening tests including hepatitis B and HIV
- hepatitis C – past or current history of intravenous drug use (IVDU) or sexual partner at high risk of hepatitis C
- alcohol use – extended liver function tests (include γ-glutamyl transferase) and where appropriate vitamin B_{12} and folate levels

Drug screening

Urine testing for drugs should be performed as part of an assessment and treatment programme. Follow-up to discuss the result should be made by the person taking the test so that the result can be relayed in the context of the history given. Refusal to consent to a drug screen may indicate some gaps or inaccuracies in the history given.

Women who disclose a past history of drug use and report that they have stopped should be offered a urine drug screen. A negative urine sample is a 'reassuring' aspect of the assessment. Women who disclose a current history of drug use should have a urine drug screen to confirm their history as part of their assessment and treatment (Table 11.3).

Harm reduction advice

Women should be given advice about the adverse effects of the specific substances they are using on the pregnancy and the baby, to facilitate informed decision making. They should also be given advice regarding the risks of the route of administration of substances; intravenous use is more risky then inhaled use, and they should be encouraged to move to a less risky route. Where injecting is ongoing, specific advice regarding the use of sterile needles, clean equipment and sharing of equipment should be given.

Table 11.3 Urine testing: detection periods for different substances

Drug	Detection period
Cannabis	2–7 days, up to 30 days if daily user
Heroin	1–2 days
Methadone	2 days
Buprenorphine	2–3 days
Benzodiazepines	1– 10 days depending on drug and usage
Cocaine	12 hours – 3 days
Amphetamines	2–3 days
Ketamine	1–4 days
Ecstasy	2–4 days

Safer sex, including the use of condoms and oral/anal sex, should be discussed. An offer of support for a substance-misusing partner should be facilitated.

Alcohol detoxification, both inpatient and outpatient, should be available to those in need. Substitute prescribing should be offered where appropriate; this will be mainly for opiate use in the form of methadone or buprenorphine (unlicensed), but may involve other substances. Substitute prescribing reduces withdrawal symptoms and avoids the risks of blood-borne virus exposure but is not risk-free. Methadone/buprenorphine dose may need to be increased during pregnancy to take account of physiological changes of plasma expansion, and methadone is often taken in split doses in the third trimester because of its increased metabolism. Slow detoxification is possible from the second trimester, but withdrawal can be complicated by miscarriage, preterm labour, fetal heart rate abnormalities and stillbirth so is not recommended.

Facilitating change

The main aim of substance misuse treatment is to facilitate change, once the patient is stable and receptive. This involves a multidisciplinary approach including a named key worker, addiction specialists and psychiatric input. For pregnant women this should be within a specialist clinic to facilitate liaison between the services and agencies involved.

Safeguarding

Safeguarding aims are twofold: to facilitate support for vulnerable families and to identify children who may be best placed with alternative carers after birth. Current substance misuse alone does not necessitate social care supervision or removal of a child; rather, the effects of the substance misuse on the woman, her partner and the home environment may require it. A Common Assessment Framework (CAF) form should be completed by the community midwife detailing all aspects of the woman's social circumstances. This should be collated with information from other agencies in contact with the pregnant woman to assess risk and decide social care involvement.

Obstetric care

Pregnant women who misuse substances and who do not have a specific obstetric risk do not necessarily need to see an obstetrician. They do however need access to an obstetrician working within the multidisciplinary team who understands their unique needs and can provide individualized care where needed. The following risk factors should be assessed to ensure safe and effective care.

VENOUS DAMAGE AND THROMBOEMBOLIC DISEASE

Women with current or past IVDU may have damaged veins, which can lead to difficulty obtaining blood samples, poor venous access, infection (see below) and thromboembolic disease (TED).

Some women will have veins damaged to such an extent that it is not possible to take blood from small peripheral veins or gain venous access for fluid resuscitation. Where veins are sparse, capillaries or femoral veins may be the only option for routine blood sampling, or it may help to 'preserve' a single patent peripheral vein for emergency intravenous access. Where venous sampling is difficult, samples may need to be prioritized and it may take several visits to complete even the bare minimum such as full blood count, blood-borne viruses and blood transfusion service samples. Some women will not tolerate venepuncture, owing to its provoking extreme anxiety associated with an anticipation of getting a 'fix' which cannot be fulfilled. Topical anaesthetic can sometimes help alleviate these symptoms.

Some patients may require central venous catheterization to achieve safe reliable venous access for delivery and/or haemorrhage. The potential life-threatening consequences of failed access need to be discussed with the woman antenatally.

The woman should have an assessment of her veins by an anaesthetist, and a plan should be made for both sampling and access. Ultrasound may aid with the identification of patent veins.

Clinicians should have a high index of suspicion for TED in this group, with a low threshold for treatment and liaison with a haematologist. Diagnosis of TED is often difficult because of the radiographic appearance of venous damage from a previous clot.

Management
- liaison with obstetric anaesthetic service
- plan for obtaining routine blood tests and venous access
- TED risk assessment at booking, at admission and postnatally
- liaison with haematology service
- harm reduction: reduce injecting

BLOOD-BORNE VIRUSES AND SEPSIS

Universal screening for BBVs should be extended for women with past or ongoing IVDU to include hepatitis C testing. Advice regarding safer sex and cervical smears should also be given.

Where the woman is hepatitis B negative she should be offered vaccination.

Where the woman is hepatitis C negative and risk is ongoing, further testing should be offered postnatally. Women who are found to be hepatitis C positive for the first time should be referred to specialist services for assessment and further treatment.

The risk of transmission of hepatitis C to the fetus during pregnancy is low, probably less than 5%. There is also a low risk of transmission during invasive testing such as chorionic villus sampling, amniocentesis or cordocentesis, and women should be counselled regarding this when appropriate. The mode of delivery should be dictated by general obstetric considerations. Fetal blood sampling should be avoided during labour. The risk of transmission during breastfeeding is negligible, and breastfeeding should be encouraged.

Women who inject drugs are at particular risk of sepsis. In the 2006–08 CMACE report sepsis was associated with six of the 35 maternal deaths related to substance misuse.[1] The use of non-sterile needles, poor veins and faulty technique contribute to the development of injection site abscesses particularly of the neck and groin. Where venous access is particularly poor, women may resort, either by accident or purposefully, to injecting into the subcutaneous skin layer, so-called 'skin popping'. When stimulants are used in this way a crater of necrotic tissue develops due to the intense vasospasm caused by the agent.

There is a tendency for clinicians to assume that symptoms in pregnant women who misuse substances are due to the substances they misuse. This tendency may lead to misdiagnosis, as highlighted in two of the 35 deaths in CMACE.[1] As with thromboembolic disease, clinicians should have a higher degree of suspicion and a lower threshold for investigation of suspected sepsis, including liaison with other specialties, in this high-risk group.

Management

- BBV testing, including hepatitis C
- hepatitis B vaccination
- liaison with specialist hepatitis services
- liaison with paediatric services
- advise partner testing for BBVs and vaccination
- inspect injection sites
- investigate for sepsis, bacterial endocarditis
- harm reduction advice – reduce injecting, aseptic technique, sharing equipment, safer sex, cervical smear

PLACENTAL PROBLEMS AND PRETERM DELIVERY

A range of placental problems are more common in this group, such as placental insufficiency and placental infarction leading to FGR, abruption and stillbirth. The cause of these problems, however, is not straightforward. Women should receive individual risk assessment and, where risks are identified, serial growth scans should be arranged. Aspirin should be considered if previous growth restriction has been severe or where there is a significant risk of concomitant hypertensive disease.

Specific obstetric risk factors affect these women in the same way as other groups. In addition, this group has a high prevalence of tobacco smoking, poor nutrition and complex social factors which also increase the risk of FGR and preterm delivery.

Stimulant drugs such as amphetamines and cocaine can cause intense vasospasm of the placental bed leading to infarction, placental insufficiency, FGR, preterm delivery, abruption and stillbirth. Alcohol, where it causes FAS or FASD, is associated with FGR, but this is not necessarily due to a direct placental effect. Alcohol is associated with preterm delivery, as is heroin, but whether this is a direct effect of the substance misuse is uncertain. Screening for preterm delivery, particularly the risk of cervical incompetence, should be carried out in the same way as for the general obstetric population.

Management
- serial scans where risk factors are identified
- consider aspirin 75 mg daily from 12 weeks
- liaise with specialist drug and alcohol services
- harm reduction advice – avoid/reduce stimulants and alcohol, smoking cessation support

MENTAL HEALTH PROBLEMS

Mental health problems affect the majority of women who misuse substances, with a significant number suffering from major psychiatric disorders such as schizophrenia, bipolar disease or borderline personality disorder. Depression, anxiety and self-harm are also common.

Where women are stable in treatment they should usually continue on their current psychiatric management even though this may include newer drugs where there is less or uncertain evidence of safety in pregnancy, as the risks of instability with discontinuation are far greater. Close liaison with psychiatric services is important to optimize safe and effective care.

Management
- usually continue current psychiatric management
- liaise with specialist psychiatric services
- harm reduction advice – continue current drug regime, inform regarding effects of illicit drugs on mental health

COMPLEX SOCIAL FACTORS

Women who misuse substances can lead lives which revolve around the acquisition of money to purchase drugs, the taking of drugs once purchased, being intoxicated followed by withdrawal symptoms and cravings. This can leave little time for essentials such as eating, financial stability, maintaining social relationships or attending for antenatal care or other appointments, for example with a social worker. Professionals describe this situation as 'chaos'.

Chaos

- woman prioritizes drug taking and drug-seeking behaviour over her own and her unborn baby's health
- too intoxicated to maintain her own health – poor nutrition and anaemia, poor/no housing, late booking and poor attendance for care
- unemployment/poor allocation of finance leads to lack of finances to maintain health – food, shelter, travel to attend for care
- relationship issues – domestic violence, sexual exploitation
- forensic issues – acquisitional, drugs, prostitution
- safeguarding issues – poor parenting, child protection issues
- fear of social services – non-engagement/avoidant behaviour, no care at all
- poor family planning – repeated pregnancies, repeated child protection orders, low self-esteem

Management

- help prioritize health – harm reduction, stabilization, substitute prescribing, nutrition
- help prioritize/rearrange appointments
- refund transport costs/arrange transport
- financial and housing benefits
- improve housing
- safeguarding process

FAMILY PLANNING

Although last in this section, contraception is arguably the most important aspect of care. Pregnancy is the greatest destabilizing event of any woman's life. An unplanned pregnancy for an already unstable substance misuser can be a devastating event resulting in the removal of a child, from which she may never recover. The offer of safe and effective contraception to all women who misuse substances has the potential to improve the health of this group of women significantly. No opportunity should be missed, including the first antenatal visit. Be positive about her upcoming baby but ask, gently, if she had thought about when she would like her next child. A timely, sensitive enquiry may be all she needs to avoid an unwanted pregnancy and all its consequences in the future.

Management
- offer family planning advice at booking
- agree method of contraception before delivery
- provide contraception before discharge home postnatally

Planning intrapartum and postnatal care

INTRAPARTUM CARE

The plan for intrapartum management should be documented antenatally. Women who misuse substances should, in general, have the same choices in labour as women who do not:

- Continuous fetal heart rate monitoring (risk of FGR).
- Pain relief choices are the same, larger doses of opiates may be required.
- Avoid cyclizine due to its potentiating the effects of opiates and its hallucinogenic properties.
- Continue methadone as prescribed.
- Fetal blood sampling is contraindicated in the presence of BBVs.
- Do not give naloxone for neonatal resuscitation; rapid withdrawal is associated with increased perinatal morbidity and death.

POSTNATAL CARE

The plan for postpartum management should be documented antenatally. Women who misuse substances should be kept together with their infants unless medical problems arise, and breastfeeding should be encouraged unless there are specific contraindications such as HIV or major antipsychotic drugs. The woman and her baby should stay in hospital for a minimum of 5 days post-delivery for monitoring of NAS symptoms and assessment and promotion of parenting skills.

Neonatal and infant problems

Neonates can suffer from withdrawal from certain substances: they may be more irritable, and are more likely to have problems feeding and interrupted sleep patterns. Breastfeeding potentiates NAS symptoms and can reduce the need for medical treatment such as oral morphine. The timing and length of NAS symptoms depends on the substances used; it is thought to be dose-dependent, but not always, and may last several weeks or longer.

Women who misuse substances have an increased risk of sudden infant death syndrome – this is strongly associated with smoking, which is more prevalent in this group. There is, however, also an association with opiates.

Table 11.4   Outline of perinatal care principles

Pre-conception care	Stabilization
	Smoking cessation
	Contraception and cervical smears
	Folic acid, vitamin D, healthy diet
	Rubella and BBV testing
	Smoking cessation
Community booking appointment 10/40	Identification of current substance misuse
	Referral to specialist midwife team
	Urine drug screen for past drug use; if positive, refer to specialist midwife team
Substance misuse antenatal care 12/40	Comprehensive assessment of substance misuse
	Assessment of social circumstances
	Assessment of comorbid medical conditions
	Obstetric risk assessment
	Advice regarding risks of substance misuse
	Discuss contraception
	Targeted aspects:
	• Advice re IVDU
	• Inspect veins
	• Hepatitis C testing
	• Extended LFTs
	• Alcohol detoxification
	• Substitute prescribing
	Referral to/liaise with appropriate specialist services/agencies
	Plan of care for antenatal, intrapartum and postpartum periods
16/40	Feedback results and plan management accordingly
20/40	Multi-agency safeguarding meeting and referral to social care if appropriate
28/40	Growth scan if risk factors
	Child protection case conference
32/40	Growth scan if risk factors
	Anaesthetic review
	Discuss and agree contraception
36/40	Growth scan if risk factors
	Home visit
	Discuss care of baby with NAS/FAS
Postnatal	5-day stay
	NAS observations
	Feeding plan
	Parenting support for mother and father
	Implement contraceptive plan
	Liaise with other services/agencies regarding discharge

Maternal health

Routine advice should be given regarding cervical smears and contraception.

Women who are receiving substitute prescription with either methadone or buprenorphine can often tolerate a reduction in their dose of 5%, and this should be discussed.

Key summary points

- Attitude – A non-judgemental supportive attitude of healthcare professionals promotes engagement of women with substance misuse, thus improving outcomes.

- Hidden harm – There should be routine use of good screening tools to identify women antenatally.

- Holistic coordinated care – The specialist midwife should coordinate the care, ensuring liaison with other specialties and services.

- Safeguarding – There should be processes in place to ensure safeguarding of the mother, her unborn child and any other children.

- Contraception – Family planning should be an integral part of services to optimize long-term outcomes for mother and baby.

References

1. Cantwell R, Clutton-Brock T, Cooper G, *et al.* Saving Mothers' Lives: reviewing maternal deaths to make motherhood safer: 2006–2008. The Eighth Report of the Confidential Enquiries into Maternal Deaths in the United Kingdom. *BJOG* 2011; 118 (Supplement 1): 1–203.

2. World Health Organization. *International Statistical Classification of Diseases and Related Health Problems*, 10th revision (ICD-10). http://www.who.int/classifications/icd/en (accessed 28 July 2015).

3. Department of Health (England) and the devolved administrations. *Drug Misuse and Dependence: UK Guidelines on Clinical Management.* London: Department of Health (England), the Scottish Government, Welsh Assembly Government and Northern Ireland Executive, 2007.

4. National Institute for Health and Care Excellence (NICE). *Pregnancy and Complex Social Factors: A Model for Service Provision for Pregnant Women with Complex Social Factors.* NICE Clinical Guideline CG110. London: NICE, 2010.

Further reading

Department for Skills and Education. *The Common Assessment Framework for Children and Young People. Practitioner's Guide: Integrated Working to Improve Outcomes for Children and Young People.* London: DfES, 2006.

Whittaker A. *The Essential Guide to Problem Substance Use During Pregnancy: A Resource Book for Professionals*, 3rd edn. London: DrugScope, 2011.

12 Screening for fetal anomalies

Dilly Anumba

Introduction

Up to 3% of pregnancies are affected by fetuses with structural anomalies. A proportion of these fetuses will have an underlying chromosomal defect. An important aspect of prenatal care is to enable pregnancies to be screened for such defects, thus providing women with choices regarding care, optimizing place of delivery and assembling the care team with the relevant expertise to provide the best care for mother and baby. Over the last few decades screening for fetal structural abnormalities and aneuploidy have therefore become cardinal components of antenatal care.

Since the introduction of ultrasonography in the 1970s there have been great strides and advancements that enable better visualization of fetal anatomy, as well as improved protocols for the evaluation of the fetus for structural anomalies. This has led to the use of ultrasound not only for dating pregnancies and the detection of multiple pregnancies, but also for the identification of the majority of serious fetal anomalies. With adequate training and quality control, high detection rates can be achieved by ultrasonography. In many parts of the developed world the routine anomaly scan is now offered to all pregnant women, usually in mid-trimester around 18–21 weeks gestation.

The principles and modalities of prenatal screening for fetal structural and chromosomal abnormalities are discussed in this chapter.

Screening for structural anomalies

Ultrasound screening for fetal anomalies is routinely offered in the UK between 18 weeks 0 days and 20 weeks 6 days. However, there is an increasing move towards the detection of the major fetal abnormalities before this time, optimally at the time of a scan between 11 and 14 weeks gestation. Earlier detection of anomalies enables women to make decisions regarding their pregnancies at an

Antenatal Disorders for the MRCOG and Beyond, Second Edition, ed. Dilly Anumba and Shehnaaz Jivraj.
Published by Cambridge University Press. © Cambridge University Press 2016.

earlier time, when pregnancy termination may be offered by medical as well as surgical means and before women have started feeling fetal movements. Furthermore, earlier detection provides a longer window of time for referral to specialist units and for additional investigations that inform subsequent care and delivery.

At the first contact with a healthcare professional (see Chapter 1), women should be given information about the purpose and implications of the anomaly scan to enable them to make an informed choice as to whether or not to have the scan. The purpose of the scan is to identify fetal anomalies and allow:

- reproductive choice (termination of pregnancy)
- parents to prepare (for any treatment/disability/palliative care/termination of pregnancy)
- managed birth in a specialist centre
- intrauterine therapy

Women should be informed that some of the major anomalies may be seen at the time of the first-trimester dating scan, but that the majority of structural abnormalities are more likely to be detected on a routine structural survey performed at 18–21 weeks gestation. They should be also informed of the limitations of routine ultrasound screening, and that detection rates vary by the type of fetal anomaly, the woman's body mass index and the position of the unborn baby at the time of the scan.

DIAGNOSTIC VALUE OF THE ROUTINE SCAN DURING PREGNANCY

Given that this practice is routine in many developed countries of the world, there is considerable evidence regarding the value of this screening assessment during pregnancy. This evidence has been recently systematically reviewed.

A recent review by NICE and the National Collaborating Centre for Women's and Children's Health (NCC-WCH) of 17 studies, including randomized controlled trials (RCTs) and prospective and retrospective studies, reported that the sensitivity and specificity of detecting fetal structural anomalies before 24 weeks of gestation reported from the included studies were 24.1% (range 13.5–85.7%) and 99.92% (range 99.40–100.00%) respectively, while overall sensitivity and specificity were 35.4% (range 15.0–92.9%) and 99.86% (range 99.40–100.00%), respectively.[1] Meta-analysis of likelihood ratios showed positive and negative likelihood ratios before 24 weeks of 541.54 (95% CI 430.80–680.76) and 0.56 (95% CI 0.54–0.58), respectively. Meta-analysis of likelihood ratios showed overall positive and negative likelihood ratios were 242.89 (95% CI 218.35–270.18) and 0.65 (95% CI 0.63–0.66), respectively.

When these studies were assessed by criteria adopted by a Royal College of Obstetricians and Gynaecologists (RCOG) workgroup, ultrasound performed before 24 weeks gestation appeared to demonstrate detection rates for anomalies likely to be lethal of 83.6%, for anomalies associated with possible survival and long-term morbidity of 50.6%, for anomalies amenable to intrauterine therapy of 100% (but $n = 3$), and for anomalies associated with possible short-term immediate morbidity of 15.5%.[2]

Taken together, these studies, which were conducted across Europe and the United States, showed that second-trimester ultrasound demonstrates high specificity but poor sensitivity for identifying fetal structural anomalies, good summary value for positive likelihood ratio but poor negative likelihood ratio. However, the values reported in the assessed studies varied widely by centre and condition.[1]

Few studies have examined routine anomaly screening in the first trimester in low-risk pregnancy populations, most data emanating from tertiary units managing high-risk pregnancies. One study published in 1999 was a prospective cross-sectional study at a university hospital in the UK, and included 6634 unselected women carrying 6443 fetuses. All women underwent either transabdominal or transvaginal sonography at 11–14 weeks. The study reported that incidence of anomalous fetuses was 1.4%, and sensitivity (detection rate) was 59.0% (37/63 (95% CI 46.5–72.4%). The specificity was 99.9%. Positive and negative likelihood ratios were 624.5 and 0.41 respectively. Although good-quality data are limited, this study suggested that the high specificity and positive likelihood ratio reported were moderated by modest sensitivity and negative likelihood ratio.[3]

In terms of clinical effectiveness, a systematic review has demonstrated that routine ultrasound screening for fetal anomalies is associated with improved pregnancy dating, detection of fetal abnormality, a threefold increase in termination of pregnancy for fetal abnormality (OR 3.19, 95% CI 1.54–6.60), and reductions in the number of undiagnosed twins and inductions for 'post-term' pregnancy.[1] No studies have as yet demonstrated improved long-term pregnancy outcomes, or any evidence of improved effectiveness of a routine first-trimester scan for detecting major fetal malformation compared with a routine second-trimester scan.

Antenatal detection of cardiac anomalies poses particular challenges and is probably the investigation that has been shown to be improved by coordinated training aimed at extending the standard views sought – from simply the four-chamber view to including the views of the cardiac outflow tracts as well as the drainage of the pulmonary veins. Employing such extended cardiac views when screening for cardiac anomalies also appears to be cost-beneficial when compared to screening approaches limited to demonstrating solely the four-chamber view. A few studies have shown that with conditions such as transposition of the great arteries (TGA), antenatal detection can improve neonatal survival and outcome by optimizing the birth and immediate neonatal care plans. It is therefore now recommended to aim to achieve a good four-chamber view of the fetal heart and outflow tracts during the conduct of the routine anomaly scan. While raised nuchal translucency is associated with a higher prevalence of cardiac anomaly in affected fetuses, it is not recommended as part of routine screening for cardiac anomalies as its predictive accuracy is not sufficient for widespread adoption.

The practice of screening for neural tube defects by maternal serum α-fetoprotein determination has now been largely replaced by direct ultrasound visualization of the neural tube, which has the capacity to detect more than 80% of significant lesions by a combination of direct visualization of the lesion and the visualization of the so-called 'head signs' of the lemon-shaped head and the banana-shaped cerebellum during the routine anomaly san at 18–21 weeks. Thus when routine ultrasound screening is performed to detect neural tube defects, α-fetoprotein testing is not required.

Screening for Down's syndrome

In the UK all pregnant women are offered Down's syndrome screening during pregnancy. Historically the benchmark for this service has gradually shifted, to prescribe minimum standards with increasing detection rates (sensitivity) and decreasing false-positive rates. The service has evolved from screening only women at advanced maternal age to universal screening, which recognizes that the vast majority of Down's syndrome pregnancies occur in women who are below the age of 35 years, despite the rapid increase in individual risk with maternal age above 37 years. In the late 1990s and early 2000s the required test performance for the Down's syndrome screening programme was that tests offered to pregnant women should attain a detection rate above 60% and a false-positive rate of less than 5%. By April 2007, UK national standards mandated that pregnant women should be offered a screening test which provides a detection rate above 75% and a false-positive rate of less than 3%. These performance measures are required to be age-standardized with a defined predictive cut-off threshold for defining risk positivity and offering a diagnostic test.

In the UK, screening for Edwards' and Patau's syndromes is now also routinely offered in the first trimester.[4]

THE PROVISION OF DOWN'S SYNDROME SCREENING DURING ANTENATAL CARE

All pregnant women should be offered screening for Down's syndrome. Screening should start with the provision of unbiased, evidence-based information about the condition, enabling women to make autonomous, informed decisions. Ideally, this information should be made available early in the pregnancy, preferably on first contact with a healthcare professional, so that women have enough time to carefully consider the options and seek further information if needed.

Care providers involved with screening must be trained to be conversant with the screening modalities offered within their service, as well as the predictive accuracy and reliability of such techniques. They should give pregnant women information about the detection rates and false-positive rates of any Down's syndrome screening test being offered, and about further diagnostic tests that may be offered. The woman's right to accept or decline the test should be made clear. Specific information should include:

- the screening pathway for both screen-positive and screen-negative results
- the decisions that need to be made at each point along the pathway and their consequences
- the fact that screening does not provide a definitive diagnosis, and a full explanation of the risk score obtained following testing
- information about chorionic villus sampling and amniocentesis
- balanced and accurate information about Down's syndrome

If a woman receives a screen-positive result for Down's syndrome, she should have rapid access to appropriate counselling by trained staff.

Screening for Down's syndrome should be performed by the end of the first trimester (13 weeks 6 days), but provision should be made to allow later screening (which could be as late as 20 weeks 0 days) for women booking later in pregnancy. Either ultrasound or maternal serum biochemistry, or a combination of both approaches, may be employed. Table 12.1 summarizes the common screening tests employed within the National Health Service of the UK.

The 'combined test' enables early screening between 11 weeks 0 days and 13 weeks 6 days. For women who book later in pregnancy, the triple and quadruple tests appear to be the most clinically effective and cost-effective serum screening approaches and should be offered between 15 and 20 weeks. They are also particularly useful when it is not possible to measure nuchal translucency, owing to fetal position or raised body mass index. After 20 weeks it is deemed too late to offer screening tests, as test performance is not as accurate and the dilemmas of dealing with a screen-positive result late in pregnancy are quite substantial.

The routine anomaly scan (at 18 weeks 0 days to 20 weeks 6 days) should not be routinely used for Down's syndrome screening using soft markers. The presence

---

Table 12.1 Screening test approaches for Down's syndrome and their gestational timings

At 11–14 weeks
- nuchal translucency (NT)
- combined test (NT + hCG + PAPP-A)

At 15–20 weeks
- double test (hCG, uE3)
- triple test (hCG, uE3, AFP)
- quadruple test (hCG, uE3, AFP, inhibin A)

At 11–14 weeks and then at 15–20 weeks
- integrated test (combined test at 11–14 weeks, followed by AFP, uE3 and inhibin A at 15–20 weeks)
- serum integrated test (PAPP-A and hCG at 11–14 weeks, followed by AFP, uE3 and inhibin A at 15–20 weeks).

hCG, β-human chorionic gonadotrophin; PAPP-A, pregnancy-associated plasma protein A; AFP, α-fetoprotein; uE3, urinary oestriol.

of an isolated soft marker on the routine anomaly scan, with the exception of increased nuchal fold, should not be used to adjust the a priori risk for Down's syndrome. The presence of two or more soft markers on the routine anomaly scan should prompt the offer of a referral to a fetal medicine specialist or an appropriate healthcare professional with a special interest in fetal medicine. However, their performance as screening tools remains contentious and unproven in large trials.

Screening tests should generate a numerical risk of the pregnancy being affected by Down's syndrome, taking into account maternal age and gestational age. This risk or chance should then be summarized as screen-positive or screen-negative based on a nationally agreed cut-off level, determined on the basis of manpower, resource and cost–benefit considerations, which should facilitate decision making. A screen-positive result should lead to a careful discussion with the couple concerning the options for diagnostic testing by way of amniocentesis or chorionic villus sampling. The pros and cons of both approaches and the basic principles of the cytogenetic analysis employed in the local laboratory, as well as the risks of miscarriage associated with each technique, should be fully discussed with the couple. An excess risk of fetal loss of approximately 1% compared with women with no invasive testing is universally quoted, but wherever possible local figures should be used in discussion with couples.

The diagnostic accuracy results reported for first-trimester screening vary remarkably, but quality-controlled large series suggest similar detection rates that vary between 80% and 90%, at false-positive rates that vary between 3% and 5%.[1] For the quadruple biochemical test in the second trimester, diagnostic accuracy is reported to vary, with detection rates of 78–85% and false-positive rates of 2–8%. Comparable detection rates are achieved by integrated tests, but there is a 25% drop-out rate, women often having to be sent reminders to attend for the second test screen. This has raised concerns about the practicality of this approach in routine practice despite some evidence that it is equally cost-beneficial.

Down's syndrome screening has been demonstrated by several studies to be acceptable to pregnant women, and has also been shown by health-economic evaluations to be cost-beneficial. However, attaining the ideal of a cost-effective screening test with the highest detection and lowest false-positive rates remains a goal, arguably attainable by the non-invasive assessment of fetal genetic material in maternal blood obtained in the first trimester. One such approach – the assessment of cell-free fetal DNA (cffDNA) in maternal serum – holds immense promise of changing the business of screening for fetal chromosomal abnormalities, some microdeletions and other genetic defects over the coming years.

Key summary points

- Ultrasound screening for fetal anomalies should be routinely offered to pregnant women between 18 and 21 weeks gestation.

- Women should be informed of the limitations of routine ultrasound screening as well as the variation of detection rates by type of anomaly, maternal habitus and fetal position.
- If an anomaly is detected during the anomaly scan, pregnant women should be informed of the findings to enable them to make an informed choice regarding pregnancy continuation or termination.
- All pregnant women should be offered screening for Down's syndrome, performed by the end of the first trimester (13 weeks 6 days) employing the combined test or, where accurate NT assessment cannot be provided or the woman is booking late, serum screening test (triple or quadruple test) between 15 and 20 weeks.
- If a woman receives a screen-positive result for Down's syndrome, she should have rapid access to appropriate counselling by trained staff and should be offered a diagnostic test.
- The routine anomaly scan (at 18 weeks 0 days to 20 weeks 6 days) should not be routinely used for Down's syndrome screening using soft markers. However, the incidental detection of such markers (e.g. an increased nuchal fold $\geq$ 6 mm) should prompt referral to a fetal medicine specialist.

References

1. National Institute for Health and Care Excellence (NICE); National Collaborating Centre for Women's and Children's Health (NCC-WCH). *Antenatal Care: Routine Care for the Healthy Pregnant Woman*. NICE Clinical Guideline CG62. London: NICE, 2008.

2. Royal College of Obstetricians and Gynaecologists. *Recommendations Arising from the 26th Annual RCOG Study Group: Intrapartum Fetal Surveillence*. London: RCOG Press, 1998.

3. Whitlow BJ, Chatzipapas IK, Lazanakis ML, Kadir RA, Economides DL. The value of sonography in early pregnancy for the detection of fetal abnormalities in an unselected population. *Br J Obstet Gynaecol* 1999; 106: 929–36.

4. Public Health England. *Screening Tests for You and Your Baby*. London: Department of Health, 2014. www.gov.uk/topic/population-screening-programmes (accessed 3 April 2016).

Index